# 1

Spine Health Dance Therapy

## Stretching
## **Bar** Dance

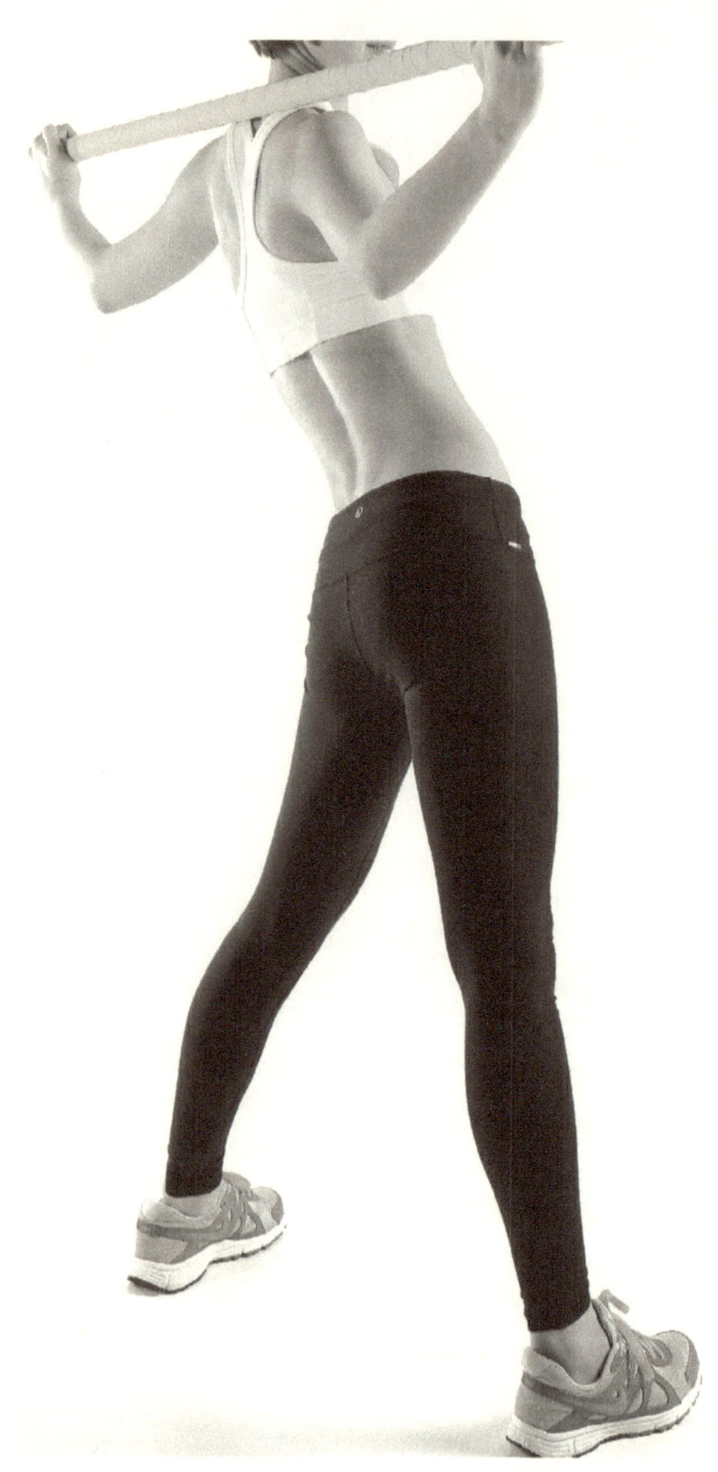

A "Stretching Bar" refers to a long stick generally used for stretching. "Stretching Bar dance" is a dance using the stretching bar designed for spinal alignment and muscle training.

Just like using a gym ball in the Gym Ball dance, which will be introduced in the following chapter, the reason for using the bar is simple. For those who are new to dancing, the most awkward parts of their body are their hands. Holding onto a bar while dancing, eliminates this problem. Also, since the bar is stiff, it helps to align posture when used in certain ways. It's like catching two birds with one stone.

# 01
# DOWN
## DANCE



We can say that the Down Dance is a full body workout that uses all muscles in the body. Disregarding age and gender, this exercise is very easy to follow for beginners because of its low level of difficulty.

This workout is also very useful in strengthening the erector spinae muscle which extends throughout the spine because the center of gravity of the body moves back when bending the knees, letting the upper body to lean back. In addition, neck and waist muscles as well as the thigh muscles, which protect and extend the knee joints, get stronger.



The Down Dance is good for those who need a full body workout but can no longer find time to exercise or have little time to exercise because of work and/or lifestyle. In addition, this full body exercise is effective for the 60-and-older seniors who can only perform a narrow range of activities due to age.



Lift the bar to the chest and stand with legs shoulder width apart.
Bending the knees, hold the core tight to prevent the buttocks from falling back. Push the bar forward, letting the upper body to lean backward slightly.
When straightening the bent knees, pull the bar towards the chest, lifting the upper body. At this moment, it is important to keep the core tight to prevent the body from swaying. You can make the movement more effective by pushing the bar strongly.

Repeat this movement 4 times.

Then, while bending and straightening the knees, stretch up the arms holding the bar overhead and lower it just above the head. Repeat the movement 4 times. In short, moving the bar forward and back 4 times and moving it up and down 4 times make a set.

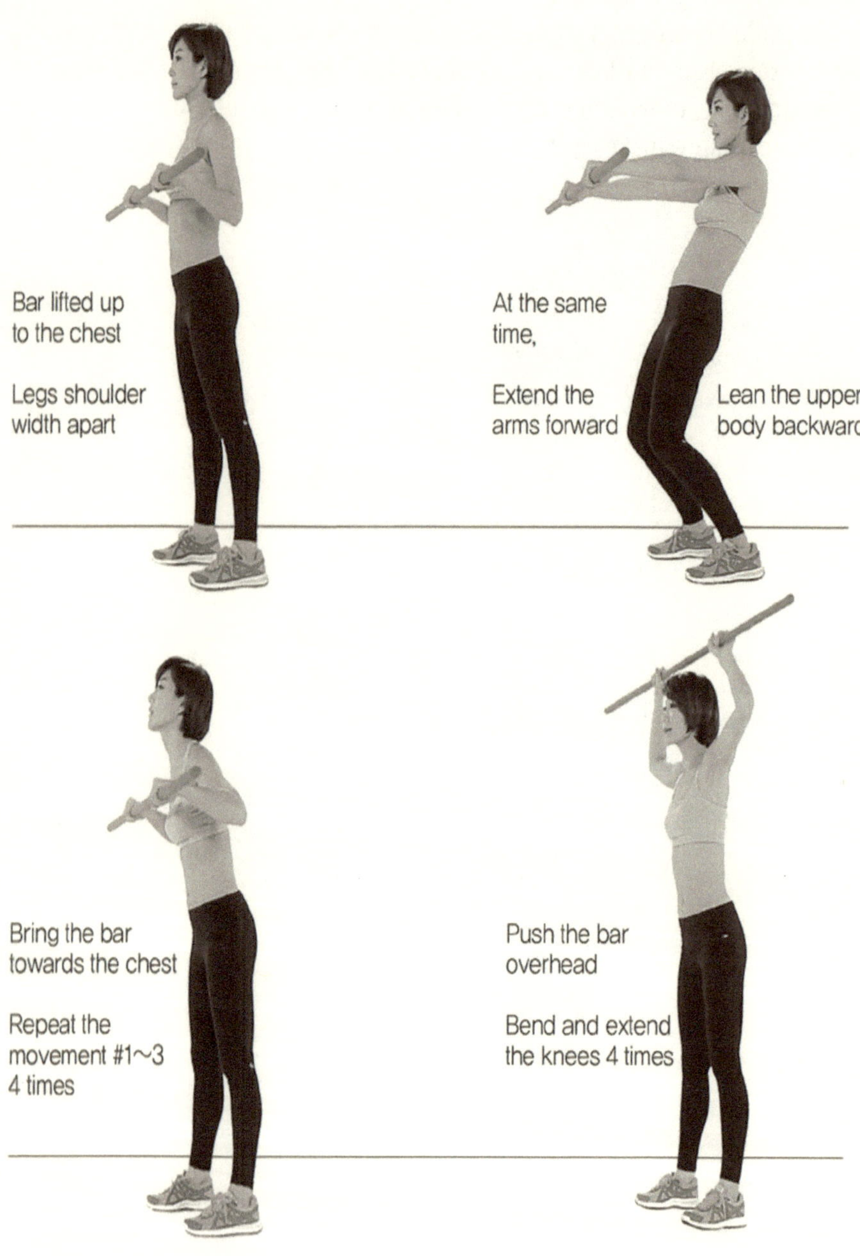


Bar lifted up
to the chest

Legs shoulder
width apart

At the same
time,

Extend the
arms forward

Lean the upper
body backward

Bring the bar
towards the chest

Repeat the
movement #1~3
4 times

Push the bar
overhead

Bend and extend
the knees 4 times

**1** Standing with the back straight and legs shoulder width apart, hold the bar with hands shoulder width apart and lift the bar up to chest level.

**2** Tightening the abdominal muscles and the lower back(the core), slightly lean the upper body backward and extend the arms pushing the bar forward.

**3** Straighten the knees and while standing upright, bring the bar towards the chest by bending your arms. Repeat the movement above 4 times.

**4** After repeating steps 2+3 4 times, bring the bar overhead, bending the knees just like in step 2. But this time, don't lean the upper body backward and keep the back straight.

**5** Straighten the knees and standing upright, bend the elbows so the bar is just above the head. Remember to keep the back straight, tightening the abdominal muscles and the lower back. Repeat steps 4+5 4 times.

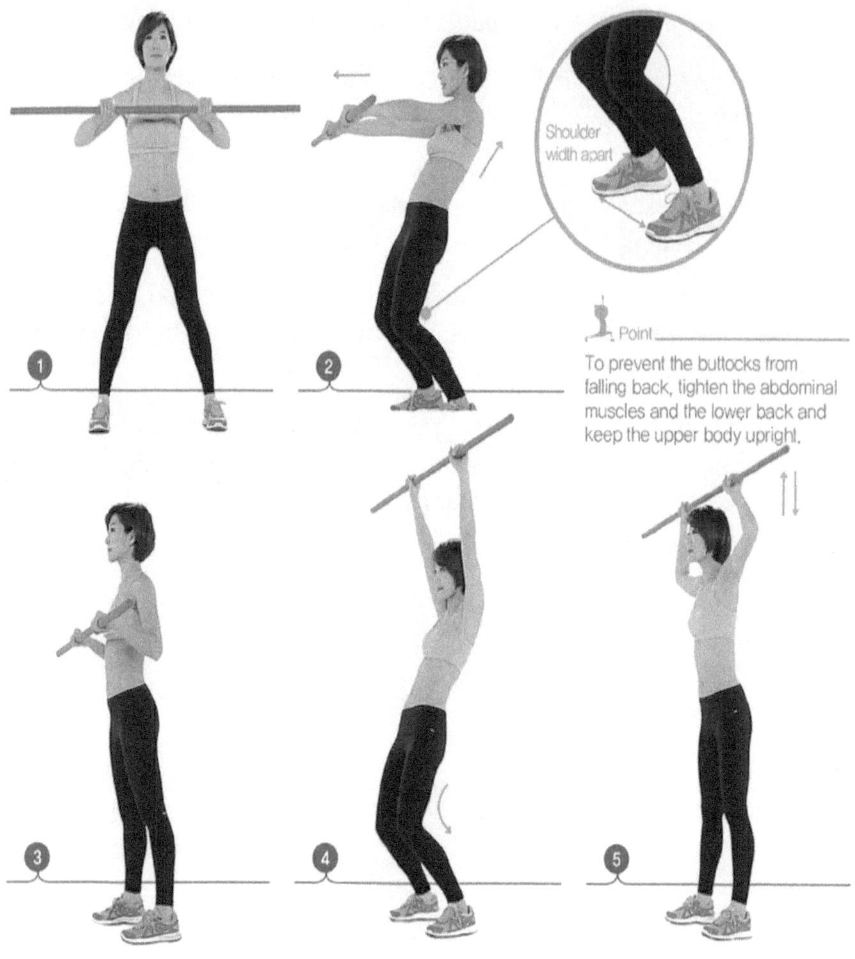




## 05 Effects

The effect that can be obtained through the Down Dance is health for the whole body. The abdominal muscles are strengthened because you basically have to tighten the stomach throughout the routine. Also, back, neck and waist muscles including the erector spinae muscle are strengthened because the upper body muscles from the waist to the neck are used when leaning the upper body back. The quadriceps femoris muscle that protects the knees is also being strengthened while bending and straightening the knees.

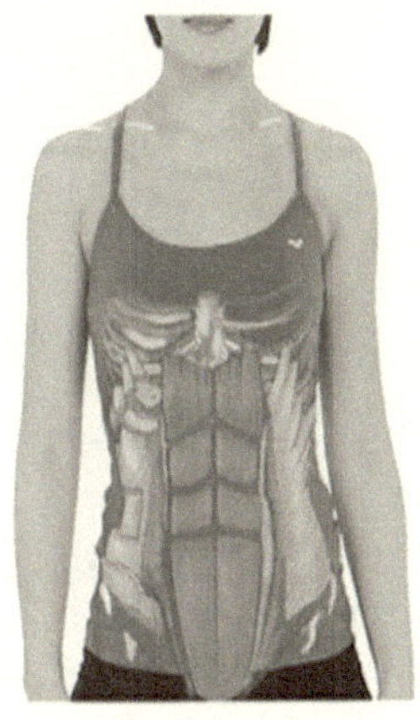

Abdominal muscles

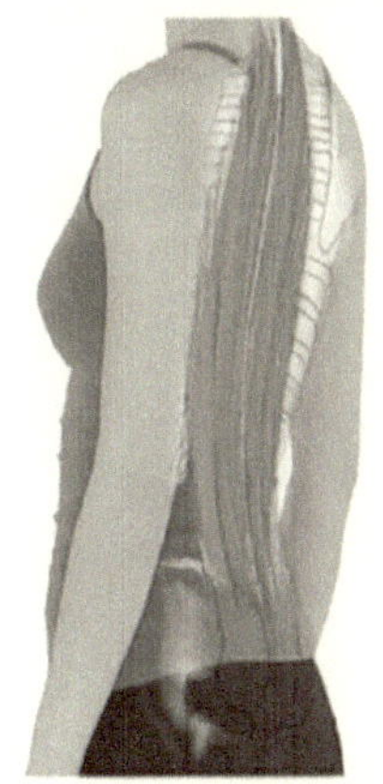

Erector spinae muscle

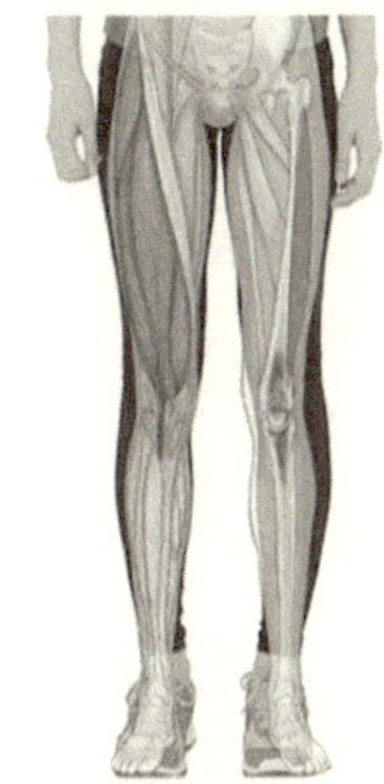

Quadriceps femoris muscle



Because the Down Dance targets all muscles, people who have had little to no physical activity may experience pain such as muscular soreness. Therefore, it is recommended to keep the beats slow at first and strengthen the muscles by repeating the movements slowly and steadily.



Mrs. K, a female in her early 40s, spends long hours sitting in front of a desk since her main job is in computer graphic design. Just like a lot of people who work long hours sitting in front of a desk, Mrs. K was a patient who experienced low back pain, shoulder and neck pain because of her poor posture.

Mrs. K has always been pushed for deadlines and so busy that she recently could not exercise. Because of her bad posture and a lack of exercise, the biggest problem for Mrs. K was that her shoulder and neck muscles were over tightened to an extent where they were causing pain.

While treating the pain, I suggested an exercise therapy, which was to slowly repeat the Down Dance movements tailored to Mrs. K's lifestyle. The first response of Mrs. K who hated any kind of exercise was a mixed feeling of helplessness and disappointment.

I continued to think that the most effective way to treat Mrs. K's repetitive pain was to strengthen her muscles through consistent exercise. We decided to see how the results turned out after a month of following the movements in the Down Dance program.

After a month, at a follow up visit, there was a noticeable difference. She no longer slouched and I noticed a healthy glow. Also, Mrs. K reported that her longtime back and neck pain were alleviated.

The Down Dance was helpful to Mrs. K, someone who hated and had little time for exercise. She could consistently exercise for about 10 to 15 minutes before going to bed wherever she was. To this day, Mrs. K completes the Down Dance exercises to exciting music for about 20 minutes every day.

Like in this case, the Down Dance allows patients to strengthen their muscles without overdoing it, naturally getting into the rhythm while dancing to exciting music.

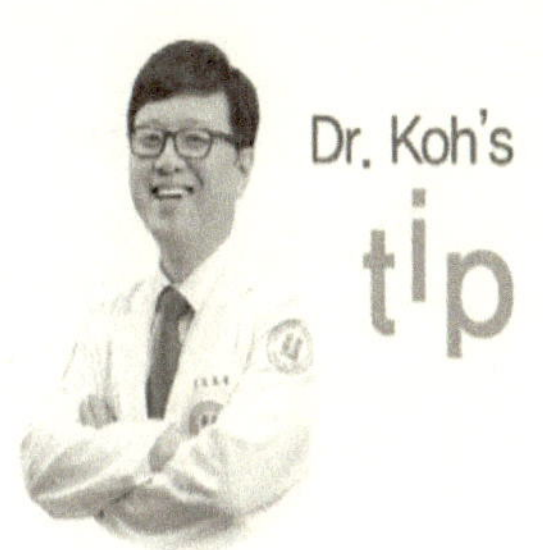


**Erector spinae muscle**

The erector spinae muscle runs along the spine vertically and plays a key role in erecting the backbone. That is why we use the word "erector" in the muscle's name. Development of this muscle is very important in order to walk upright. We have to strengthen the erector spinae muscle in order to maintain correct postures.

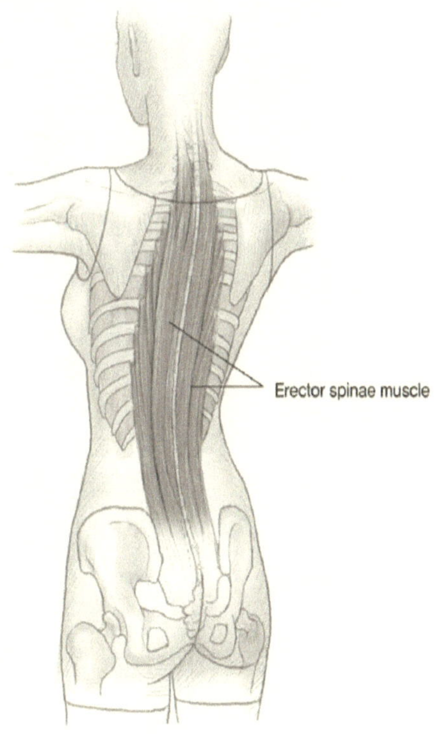

## Quadriceps femoris muscle

The quadriceps femoris muscle is a large muscle group which covers the front and sides of the thigh bone and is subdivided into four separate portions - rectus femoris, vastus lateralis, vastus medialis, and vastus intermedius. This muscle which straightens the knee joints has an important role in all leg actions including standing, walking, or running.

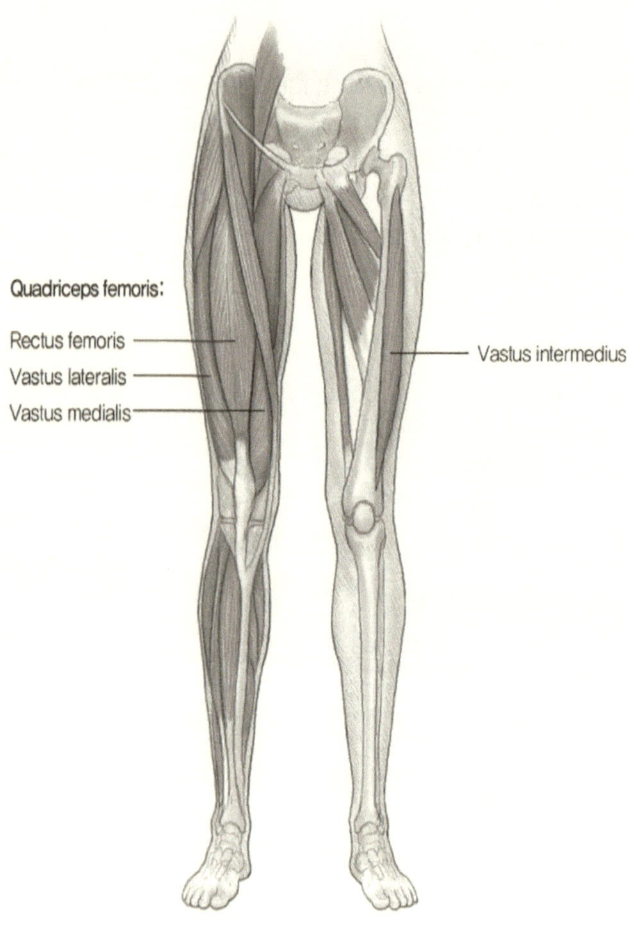

# 02
# UP
# DANCE



Up Dance is a full body workout, about four times stronger than the Down Dance. You apply twice the force while bending the knees and standing up and twice the force with alternately raising each leg.

In other words, the Up Dance is harder than the Down Dance because you work against gravity when straightening the knees after bending them. In addition, the third movement, raising one leg slightly, is twice as much difficult because all of the body weight shifts onto the other leg, activating all the muscles in the hips and the upper body.



When bending the upper body forward, you will use abdominal back, neck and waist muscles. When bending and straightening the knees, you will also use thigh muscles, making the intensity of the Up Dance much greater than the Down Dance.

Since the Up Dance is slightly more difficult than the Down Dance, it is recommended that you practice the Down Dance sufficiently and learn the rhythm before you start the Up Dance. the Up Dance is the most basic club dance.

Like the Down Dance, the Up Dance will also be a useful full body workout for those who have little to no activity. This is very effective for those who drive for long periods of time or have no power at their waist and lower body due to a sedentary lifestyle.

Standing with the back straight, bend the knees and hold the bar 12 inches away from the chest.

Then while standing up straightening the knees, slightly lean the upper body forward while holding the lower back and the legs tight. Repeat the movement twice. Remember, it is important to hold the lower back and the legs tight to prevent the buttocks from falling back.

Next, while bending and straightening the knees, raise one knee slightly outward and lean the upper body forward again. Raise each leg alternately, and repeat this movement twice.

Next, march in place for 8 counts while holding the bar at the chest. When marching in place, do not lock your knees, and keep a slight bend.

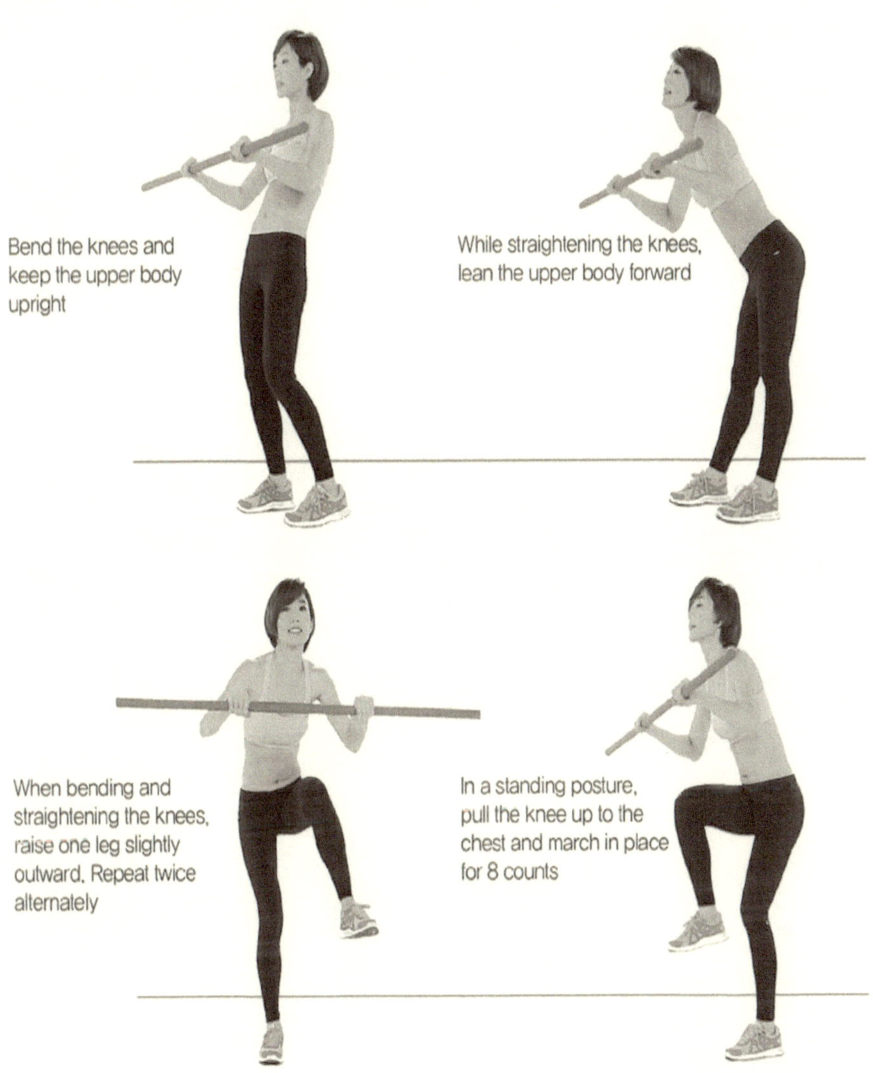


## 04 Details

**1** Bend the knees slightly to about 45 to 55 degrees and naturally place the arms holding a bar approximately 12 inches from the chest. To prevent the buttocks from falling back, hold the core tight with the back upright.

**2** While shouting "One!," strongly straighten the knees, while leaning the upper body forward, keeping the core tight to prevent the buttocks from falling back. Also, hold the lower back and the legs tight to prevent the upper body from leaning forward too far.

**3** Raise one knee as if you are pulling it towards the chest while holding the bar at the same location.

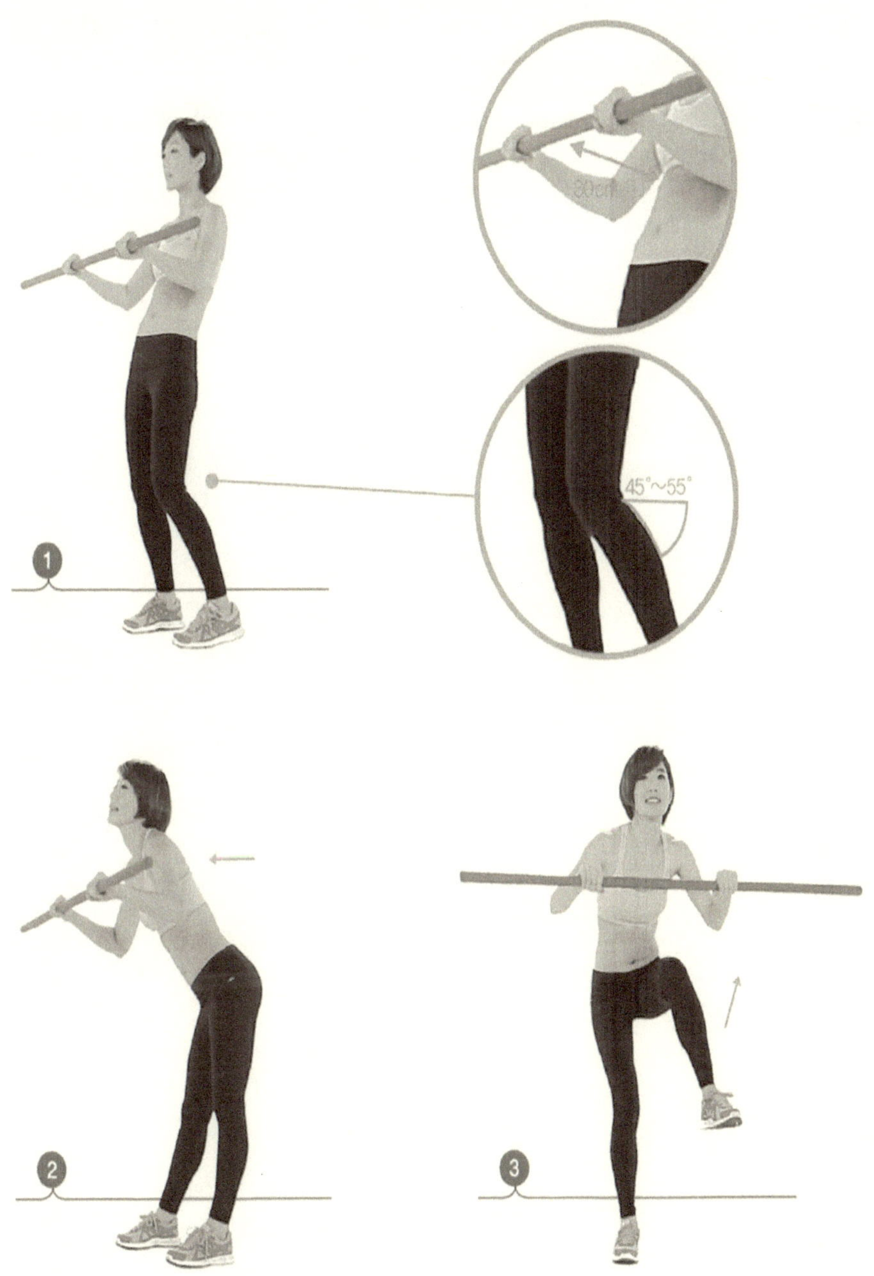


4 Lower the raised leg and lean the upper body forward, trying to prevent the buttocks from falling back just like in step #2.

5  When bending and straightening the knees again, raise the other leg towards the chest. Repeat the movement #1~5 twice.

6  Holding the bar at the same location, march in place, pulling up one knee towards the chest while slightly bending the other knee. It could be difficult at first, but you will get used to it as you repeat it for 8 counts.

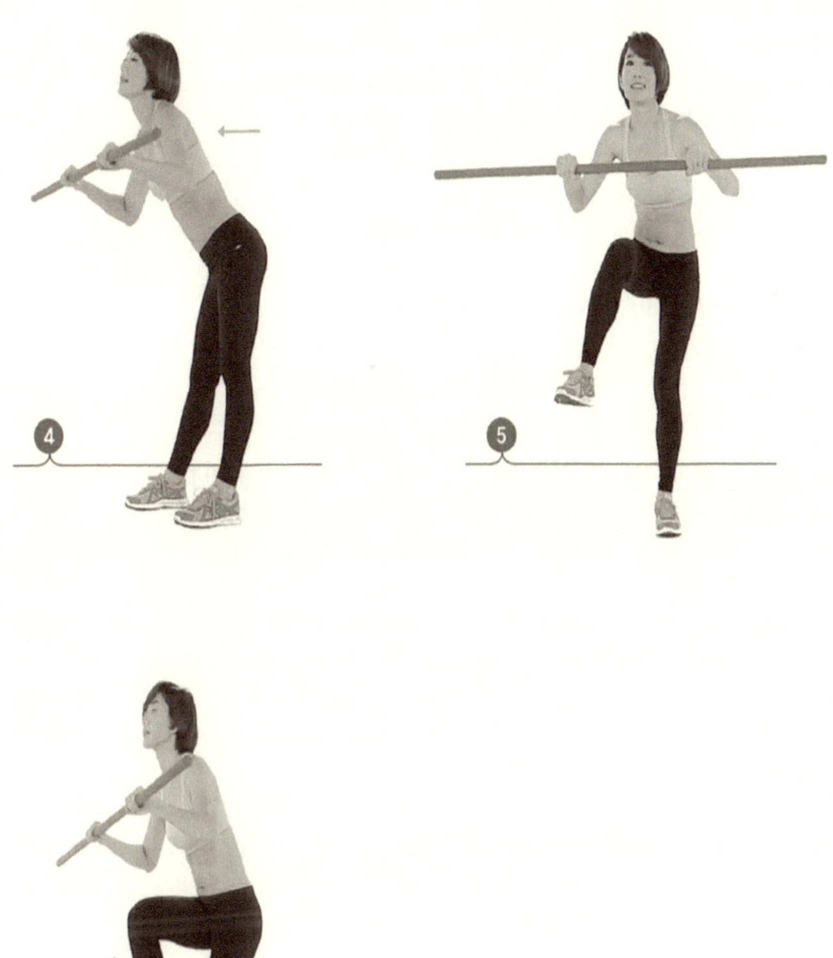

05 Effects

The biggest effect of the Up Dance is strengthening all muscles of the upper and lower body. When you straighten the knees against gravity and stand upright as you lean the upper body forward, you will use abdominal muscles, the erector spinae muscle of the back, neck and waist muscles, quadriceps femoris muscle on the front of thighs, and hamstring muscles on the back of thighs. Moreover, when raising one leg slightly, the weight of the body will shift to the other leg which activates the buttock muscles, including the gluteus medius, gluteus maximus, and others like quadratus lumborum, latissimus dorsi etc. When marching in place, you will also activate the iliopsoas and inguinal muscles. As you can see with the Up Dance, you will strengthen almost all of the muscles in the body.

 Caution

Since the workload of the Up Dance is very high compared to other kinds of dances, I advise that you try to focus on making the movements slowly and correctly until you get familiar with them before completing with faster beats.

Make sure that you stretch the neck sufficiently before the dance, as the neck muscles can get strained more often than the waist muscles in the Up Dance. (Refer to "Stretching") If you feel persistent pain in the neck even after you have stretched before dancing, it is recommended that you seek medical attention.

Everyone young and old should follow the movements one by one slowly and precisely to avoid over exertion and prevent minor muscular pain. After getting used to the movements, you will be able to dance naturally to the rhythm.

 Example

Mr. H who works in an office, is a squash enthusiast. He feels like all the stress from everyday life is gone after getting soaked in sweat as he runs back and forth, playing squash. One day, he was playing squash with one of his friends. To hit the ball, he ran as fast as he could and put all of his weight on one foot. At that moment, he felt a slight pain in his pelvis and lower back. He thought this was just a little muscle pain that comes and goes while playing squash. He did not think much of it until the pain became an obstacle in everyday life to the point where he couldn't sit or walk without pain. The result of his diagnosis showed that it was damage to the hip mucle due to intense exercise. Despite treatment, he suffered the same pain whenever the activity was intense or when he played for a slightly longer time than usual. My recommendation was to complete the Up Dance everyday.

At first, he was dubious and asked, "A dance? Would it really work?" After trying it once. He found it enjoyable and was tempted to continue. He danced the Up Dance to an overly fast beat in high intensity, which caused back pain and muscle pain all over his body. I warned that exercising too intensely too early can reduce the effect of the exercise and advised him to slow the pace and gradually increase the intensity while focusing on the accuracy of the movements. After about three months, there were significant changes in Mr. H's body.

Even though Mr. H had played squash for a long time and tried his best balancing his diet, he seemed somewhat overweight. However, three months of consistent Up Dance changed his body to look more like a trained athelete and helped him lose 12 lbs.

"At first, I couldn't feel the effects because I loosely followed the movements thinking this won't work. But when I did as Dr. Koh advised, following each movement slowly and precisely gradually increasing the pace, I realized that I started losing weight in less than a month and that the shape of my body was changing. Excited, I fervently and diligently followed the program. My physical endurance, which usually ran low by the end of the workday, stayed strong. I was surprised to find out that the dance therapy really works and I have more energy in my everyday life."

Realizing the effect of the Up Dance, Mr. H has learned the other dance movements and dances the Spine Health Dance every single day. When he recently came with his mother, who is suffering from a lower back pain, he was not the same guy I knew before. He had changed so much that I almost did not recognize him. I asked, "Is there any good news? You've completely transformed." He replied, "Thanks to you, Dr. Koh, dancing every day at home, I'm happy that I'm in good health, lost weight and gained the strength to overcome mental stress." As the creator of the Spine Health Dance, this was a truly rewarding moment for me.

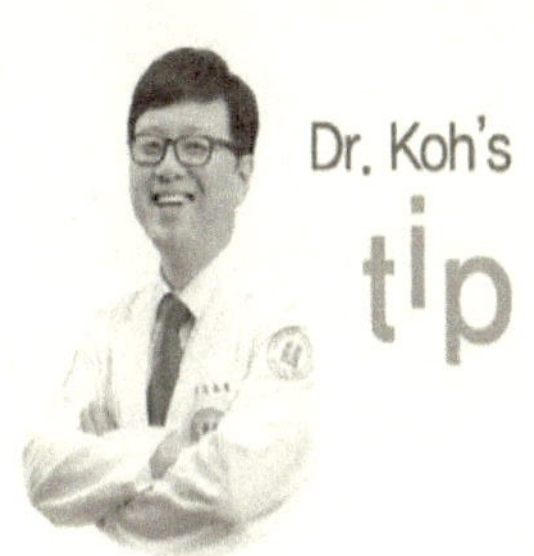


**Gluteus medius muscle**

The gluteus medius muscle covers the front, mid, and rear surface of the pelvis, stablizing the head of the femur and the pelvis. When rotating the hip joint externally, walking, or supporting the weight with one leg, this muscle holds the pelvis in place on the weight bearing side and prevents the pelvis on the opposite side from dropping too much.

Gluteus medius muscle strain can happen from standing on one leg for a long time, and or walking with bad posture. Problems with the gluteus medius muscle can cause low back pain, hip pain, and lateral and posterior thigh pain.

**Gluteus maximus muscle**

The gluteus maximus muscle is located in the back side of the pelvis (in the buttocks), is the largest one of the gluteus muscles, and is regarded as one of the strongest muscles in the human body. This area is often used for an intramuscular injection for pain relief.

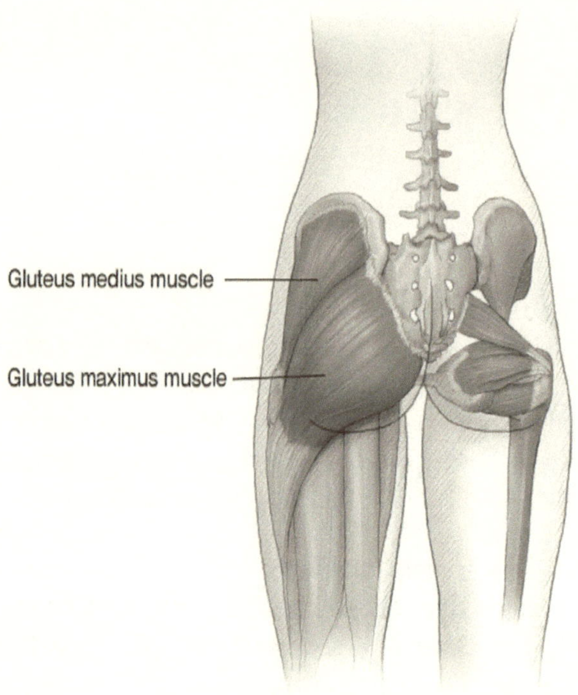



## Sacroiliac joints

The sacrum. also known as the tail bone, is an isosceles triangle shaped bone below the lumbar spine. The ilium is a fan shaped flat bone and forms the top part of the pelvis. The sacroiliac joint is the joint between the sacrum and the ilium.

The sacroiliac joint doesn't have the range of motion as compared to other joints. The sacrum and the ilium are strongly connected by the anterior and the posterior sacroiliac ligament. There is a joint gap between the two bones due to the elasticity of the ligaments, but the bones fuse with aging.

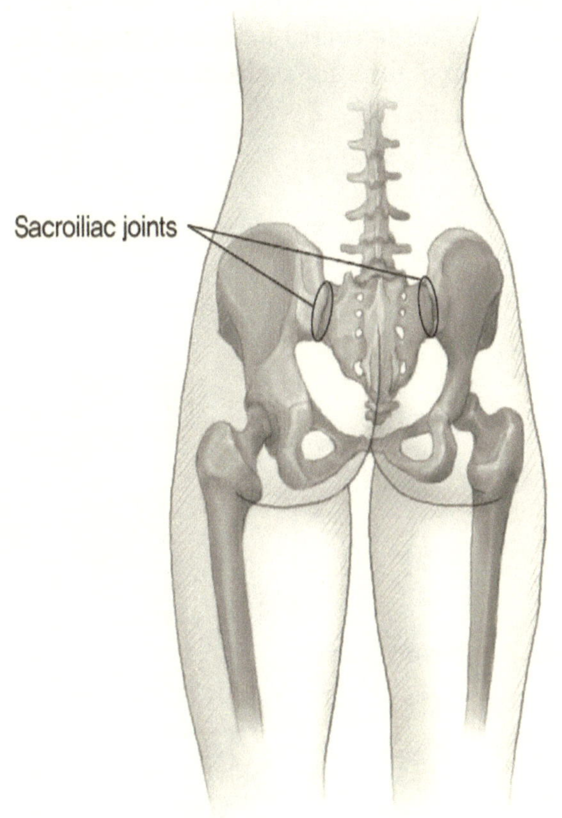



**Quadratus lumborum muscle**

The quadratus lumborum muscle is a quadrilateral shaped muscle in the waist area. This muscle runs from the iliac crest to the 12th rib and lies deep inside the posterior and lateral side of the abdomen. The outer one third region of the kidney, which is the organ in the posterior abdominal wall, lies to the muscle. The iliopsoas muscle, the inferior aspect of the posterior serratus muscle, the transversus abdominis muscle, and the erector spinae muscle are all connected to this muscle by the fascia.

Tightness in the quadratus lumborum muscle cause low back pain. If you have low back pain or hip pain for no reason or get hurt while exercising or lifting heavy stuff, the first place to look is at the quadratus lumborum muscle, also known as "the joker of low back pain." The quadratus lumborum muscle is used for side bending of the trunk and extension and rotation of the waist as the muscle is attached to the rib, the lumbar, and the ilium.

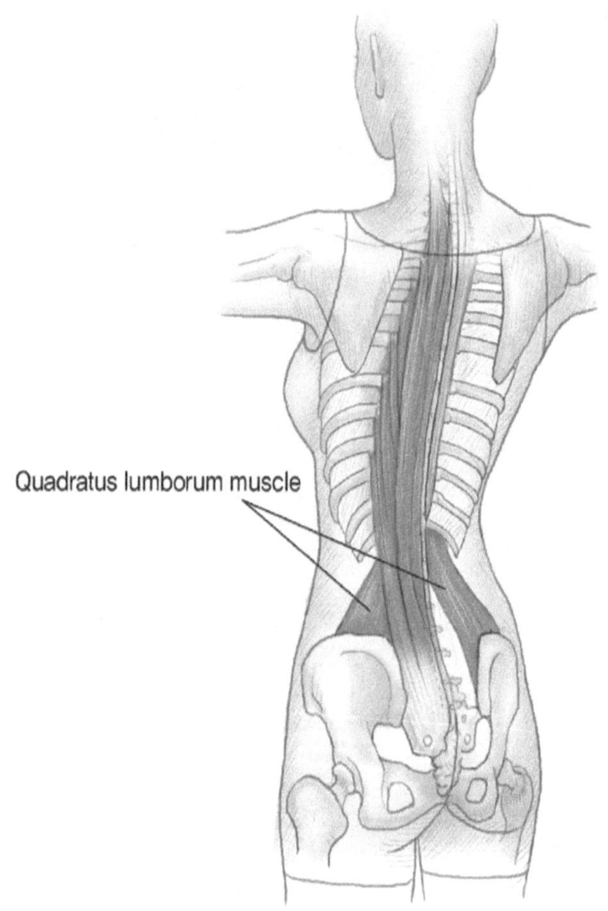



**Latissimus dorsi muscle**
The latissimus dorsi muscle starts at the bottom of the back, becomes thinner while going upward, converges to a narrow tendon, and then is attached to the humerus. This muscle is a big, flat, fan shaped muscle that spreads widely in the back. It is the widest muscle in the back. The inverted triangular body shape of swimmers come from the development

of the latissimus dorsi muscle.

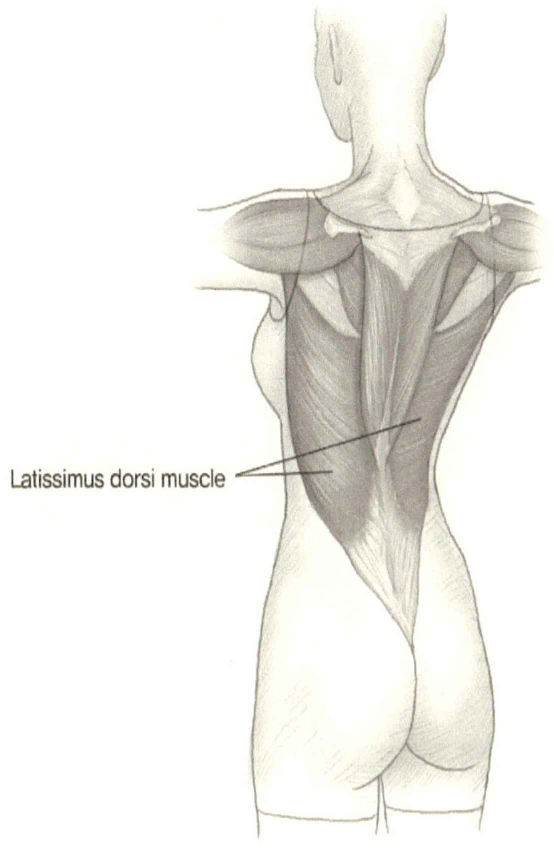



## Iliopsoas muscle

The iliopsoas muscle connects the lumbar spine to the pelvis and runs from the spine to the ilium and to the femur of the leg. One of its features is shortening from poor lifestyle habits. This can cause low back pain due to the tension of muscles, tendons and ligaments around the spine. For this reason, the spinal disc may herniate if the intervertebral disc is excessively compressed under pressure. If the iliopsoas muscle is shortened, your posture can be bent over by flexion of the pelvis and trunk, you will feel pain in the waist, pelvis and legs.

Patients can hardly stand on the affected leg and are hunched over because of low back pain caused by the iliopsoas muscle. You often see them lean forward in walking with one hand on their hip. Furthermore, they feel pain when lifting heavy weights or straightening both legs in the supine position, but they feel better when bending their legs or crouching their body in the side lying position.

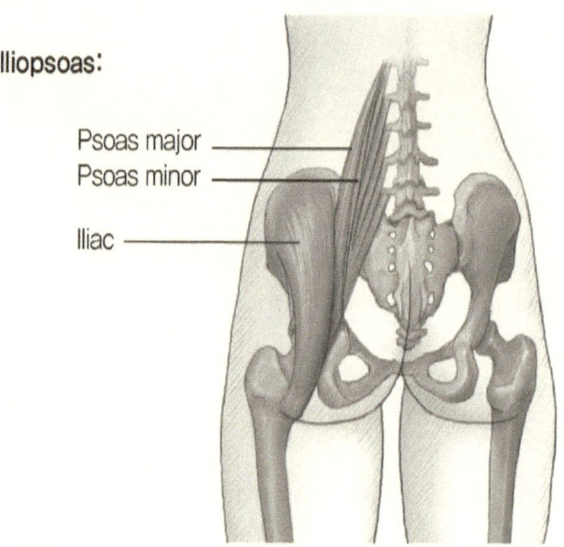



## Inguinal muscle

Lying deep inside the thigh, this muscle is often injured in athletes, those who hardly exercise to rotate their body, or those who maintain the same posture for a long period of time. To prevent the injury, it is good to strengthen the inguinal muscle (adductor muscle, pectineal muscle, and gracilis muscle).

If the inguinal muscle is injured, you feel pain in the upper thigh, especially the place where the muscle meets the pelvis in the inner thigh. In the case, it can be painful with walking, closing or spreading legs.

# 03
# **TECHNO**
# DANCE

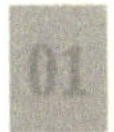 Synopsis

In the 1990s, the Techno Dance in which people repeatedly shake their neck and upper body to electronic dance music was a sensation in Korea. There were two famous celebrities at that time. Jihyun Jeon danced to techno music, wearing sexy clothes on a television commercial. Her commercial is still remembered today. The other was Jeonghyun Lee who very popular from singing and dancing to techno music.

The movements of the Techno Dance may be difficult, but the generation's ultimate dance can be a good full body workout for the spine and joints if you change a little bit of the movements. Because the Techno Dance uses the waist and the pelvis, it can help align your body and change your body shape as it uses muscles that you don't often use.

 Who needs this?

The Techno Dance can help people who are dissatisfied with their body type even though they exercise regularly, and is good for those who are not interested in weight training because they can effectively exercise to exciting music.

**03 Basic Movement**

Stand with the legs shoulder width apart and hold the bar behind the neck, placing it on the shoulders. Holding the core tight, tilting the pelvis slightly forward, push the pelvis left and right.
While moving the pelvis left and right, make sure that the knees are not bent.

keep the core tight to prevent the upper body from slouching or from leaning too far back.

After swaying the pelvis left and right twice, strongly twist the upper body in the same direction as the movement of the pelvis. At this moment, twist the neck also to turn your eyes in the same direction. It is helpful and more effective to put high rotational force in the upper body.

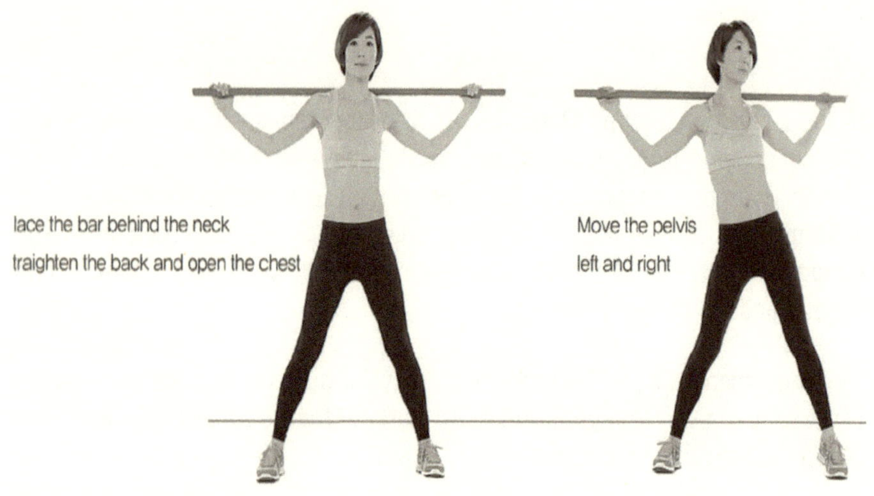



Turn the body and the neck in the direction
of the pelvic movement

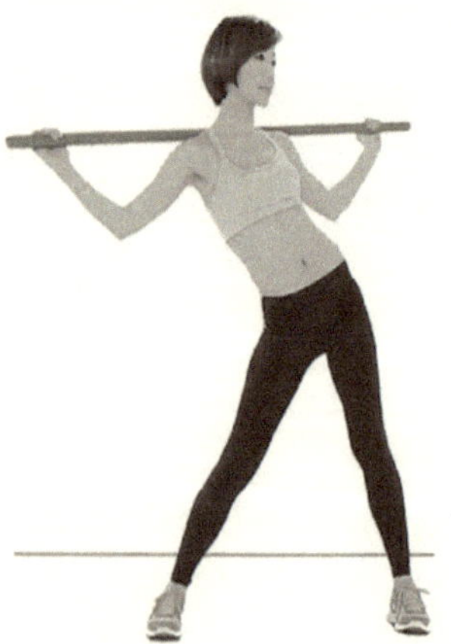

1 Stand with the legs shoulder width apart, place the bar behind the neck, and place it on the shoulders.

2 Hold the core tight, preventing the buttocks from falling back and place the center of gravity slightly backward. While maintaining this posture, sway the pelvis left and right.

3 After swaying the pelvis left and right twice, strongly turn the upper body and the neck in the direction of the pelvic movement (left).

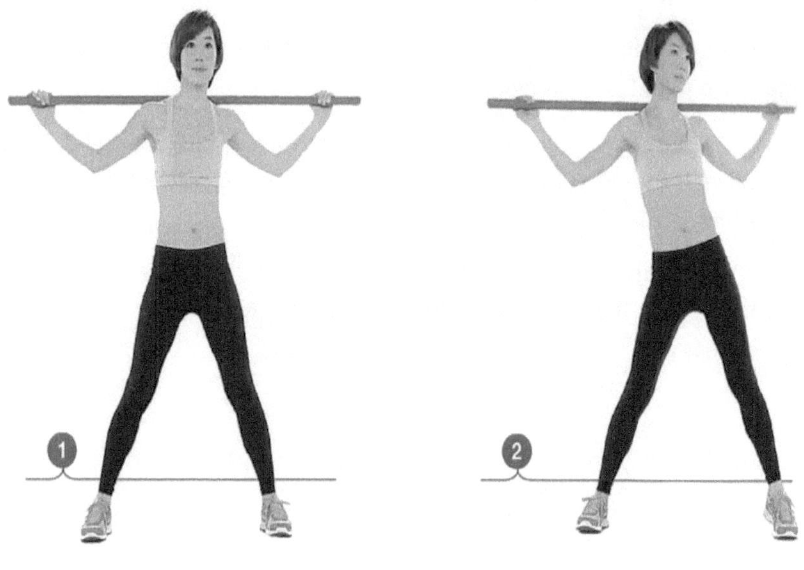

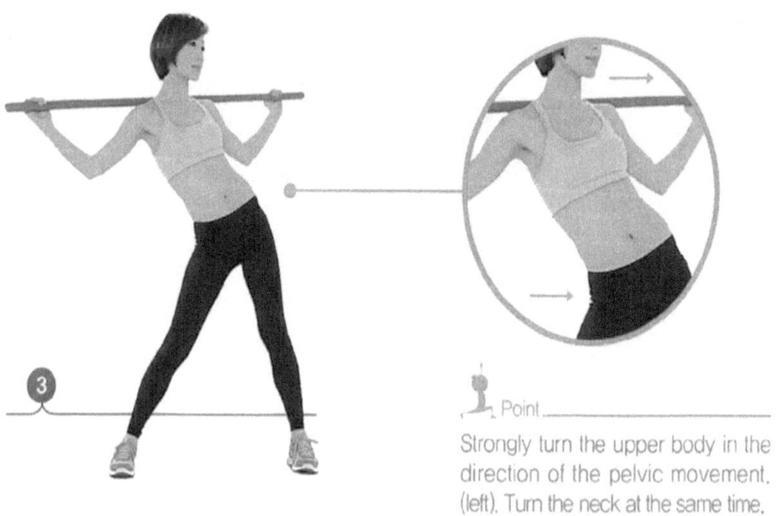



4 Then, strongly turn the upper body in the direction of the pelvic movement to the right. Turning the neck at the same time.

5 For those whose legs get numb or one side of the buttocks gets heavy after sitting for a long time, turn the upper body slightly in a smaller angle when turning the upper body in the direction of the pelvic movement. This is to prevent overloading the disc.

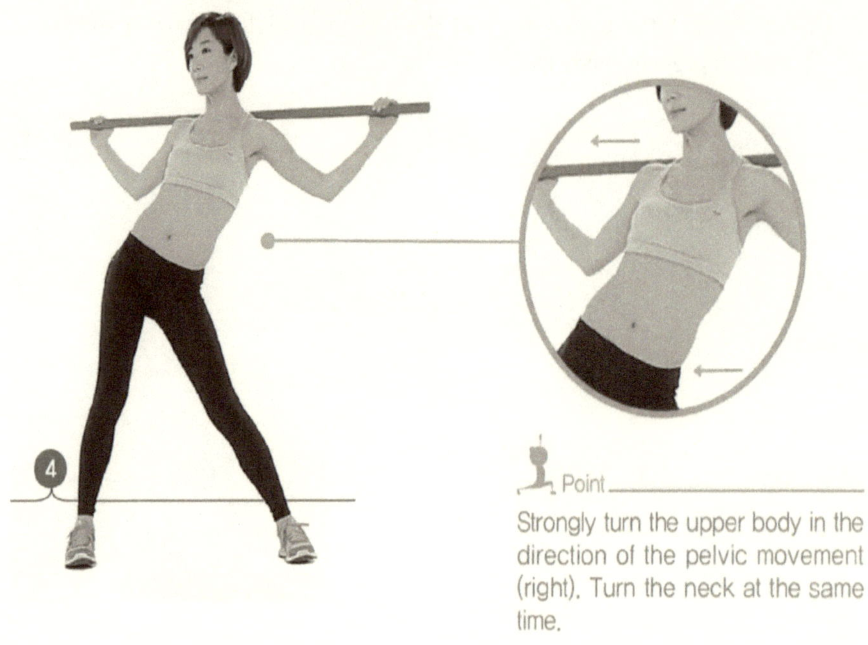



Point

Strongly turn the upper body in the direction of the pelvic movement (right). Turn the neck at the same time.

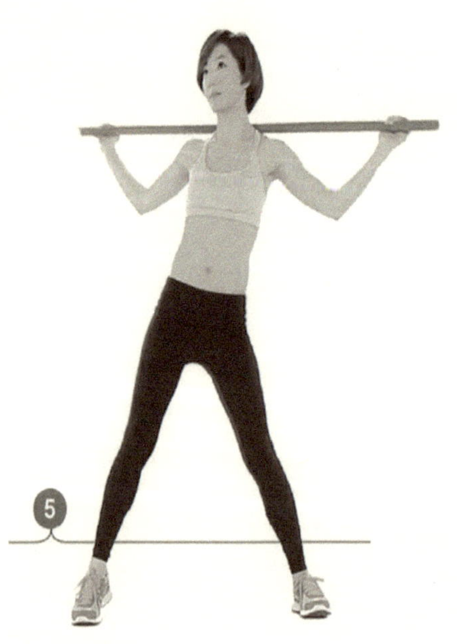

 Effects

The Techno Dance is effective for the alignment of the spine because as the pelvis moves from side to side, the waist rotates in the same direction. This will activate the oblique abdominal muscle which is usually weak, because you twist your body with the pelvis in the same direction by using the waist.

In addition, the rotation of the waist and the movement of the pelvis can make the sacroiliac joints and the deep muscles such as quadratus lumborum muscle stronger, which are often injured by lifting. The gluteus maximus and medius muscles are strengthened as you keep the feet on the ground and rotate the waist. As such, the Techno Dance aligns the body through strengthening the upper body, pelvis and hip muscles.

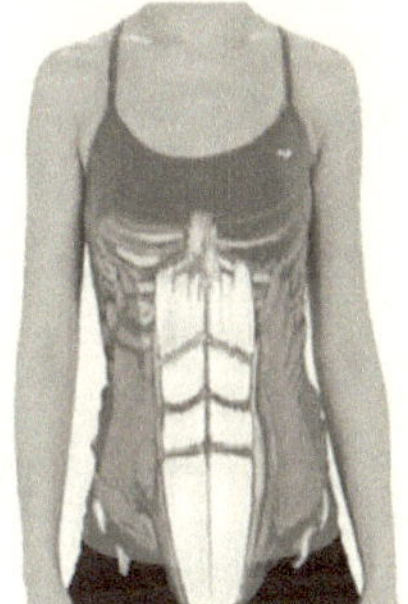 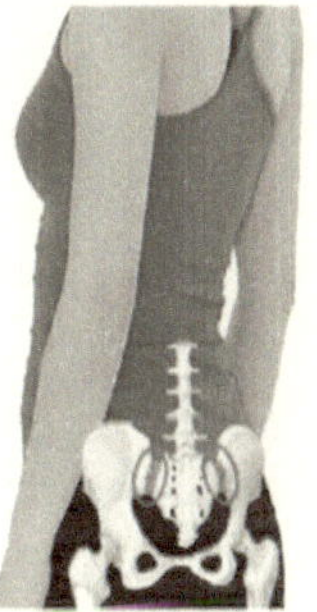 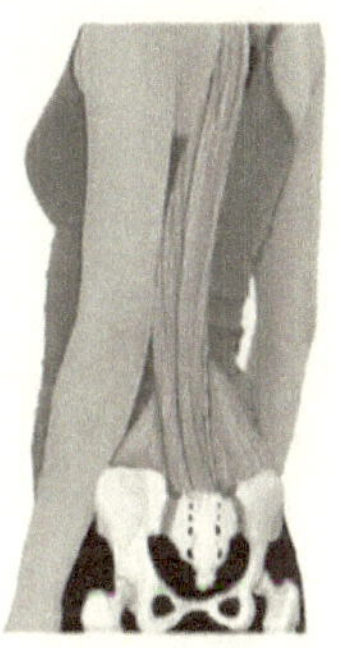 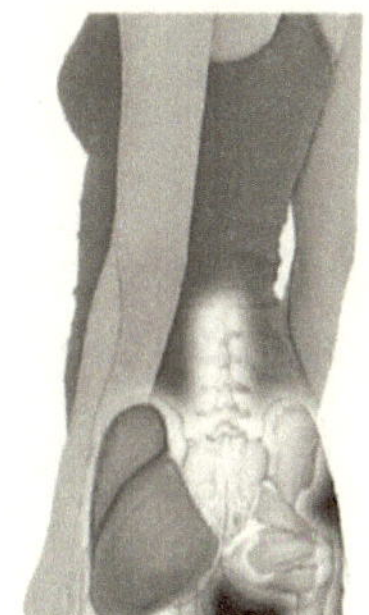

| Oblique abdominal muscle | Sacroiliac joints | Quadratus lumborum muscle | Gluteus medius (upper) and Gluteus maximus (lower) muscles |

 Caution

The main movement of the Techno Dance is the rotation using the waist and the pelvis. Older adults have to be careful when they turn their upper body and neck in the same direction because this may cause dizziness.

Vestibular organs sense horizontal and vertical alignment acceleration and rotation in the head then delivers the information to the static organs in order to control the balance of the body. For people 50 and older, the vestibular organs get weaker. Therefore, people who have a weak vestibular system shouldn't turn the neck but keep the eyes firmly fixed forward while turning the upper body in the direction of the pelvic movement.



Mr. N, a freshman in college has been my patient along with his grandmother and his parents. Mr. N has been treated for his back pain since he was a junior in high school. Scoliosis is a common spinal condition among students in their adolescence, but this was not the case for Mr. N.

Spinal conditions that appear among students are most likely due to their bad postures. There are many cases where spinal diseases are caused through straining ligaments and muscles around the neck or spine by the position of the neck to read books on a desk or slouching while sitting at the edge of a chair.

Mr. N's case was similar to this. When Mr. N became a senior in high school, during the time he needed to take the college entrance exam, he came to the hospital complaining of a frequent back pain. It was a physical issue, but the mental pressure from the exam couldn't be overlooked.

I taught Mr. N the movements of Down, Up and Techno Dance for him to exercise at home during his break times while studying. Learning how to dance from a doctor! He laughed, but thought it would be interesting and fun. After the college entrance exam, Mr. N came to me for a spine checkup with a bright smile. He said, "Thanks to you, Dr. Koh, I did quite well on the exam and I'm also getting fit."

According to Mr. N's parents, even during the most stressful time, Mr. N diligently exercised not missing a single day because it was easy dancing to his favorite music. His focus level increased when he danced as a break during his studies.

Since he started the program, he became less irritated in everyday life and felt less pain while studying. He woke up in a good mood and stopped disliking his school life, which surprised his family members.

After listening to his parents, Mr. N said, "Dancing without any concerns was the only happy time for me. As time passed, those challenging days were not that tough anymore and I felt somewhat healthier. I lost a little weight and gained some muscle. I'm happy with the results. In fact, I don't feel pain in my back anymore and I don't get tired that easily when I play basketball with my friends."

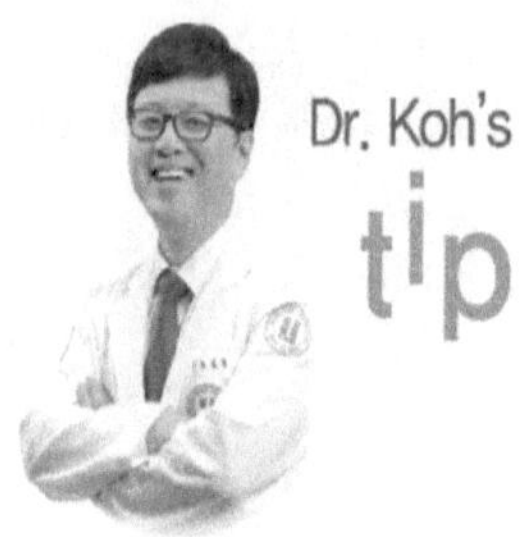


### Oblique abdominal muscle

The oblique abdominal muscles consists of the external oblique muscle and the internal oblique muscle. The external oblique muscle runs in the same direction as the external intercostal muscle and the internal oblique muscle runs in the same direction as the internal intercostal muscle. In other words, the muscle that are on the lateral side of the abdominal muscles is the oblique abdominal muscle.

If you put your right hand on the left side of your abdomen obliquely downward and then overlap your left hand on the right hand perpendicularly, your left hand describes the direction of fibers in the external oblique muscle and your right hand describes the direction of fibers in the internal oblique muscle.

When batters twist their waist and swing at the pitch or when pitchers throw a ball, they often injure their oblique abdominal muscles. An injury to the oblique abdominal muscle transmits pain diagonally downward from the xiphoid area to the costal arch or from the pubis to the costal arch. In this case, diagnosis isn't easy because the symptoms are similar to issues of internal organ problems.

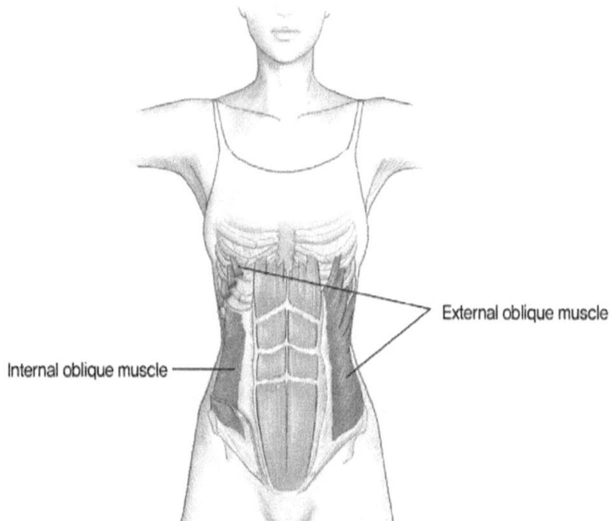

External oblique muscle
Internal oblique muscle

# 04

# ELECTRONIC
# DANCE

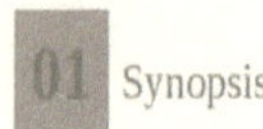 Synopsis

Electronic Dance which was popular among young people at clubs is similar to the Down Dance, but the difference in the Electronic Dance is moving the buttocks backward instead of leaning the upper body backward while bending the knees. You have to straighten the upper body and place the bar behind the waist in order to prevent the upper body from slouching while moving the buttocks backward.

The most important thing in this dance is that you don't fully extend your knees but keep them slightly bent while you bounce to the rhythm. Original electronic dance has more upper body movement, but this Electronic Dance doesn't have any upper body movement and keeps the upper body upright for consideration of the spine.

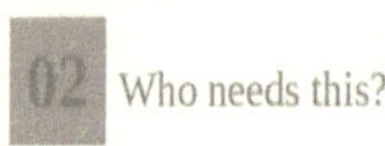 Who needs this?

The Electronic Dance is especially effective for people whose muscles surrounding the spine are weak even with steady exercise. This can help build a stronger back for patients who have low back pain without evidence of trauma or disc problems.

Even with a strong and healthy spine, this dance can help maintain a healthy body and prevent spine diseases due to aging. Also, if you want to build muscle, dancing steadily the Down Dance, the Up Dance, the Techno Dance, and the Electronic Dance together can be as effective as weight training.

Place the bar behind the waist hold onto it with both hands and stand with legs shoulder width apart. Bend and straighten the knees just like how it was done in the Down Dance. Make sure that the knees do not lock but kept slightly bent. As you are repeating this leg movement, gradually get into the rhythm.

When bending the knees, make sure to keep the upper body straight, open the chest, and slightly pull out the buttocks backward. At this moment, you would feel like the pelvis is also pulled out backward with the buttocks. The buttocks should be pulled backward as much as possible, but not to the point where you sit down.

In the rhythm, pull out the buttocks backward when bending the knees. straighten the knees until it is still slightly bent and place the buttocks to the original position. Again, pull out the buttocks backward, bending the knees. Repeat this movement.

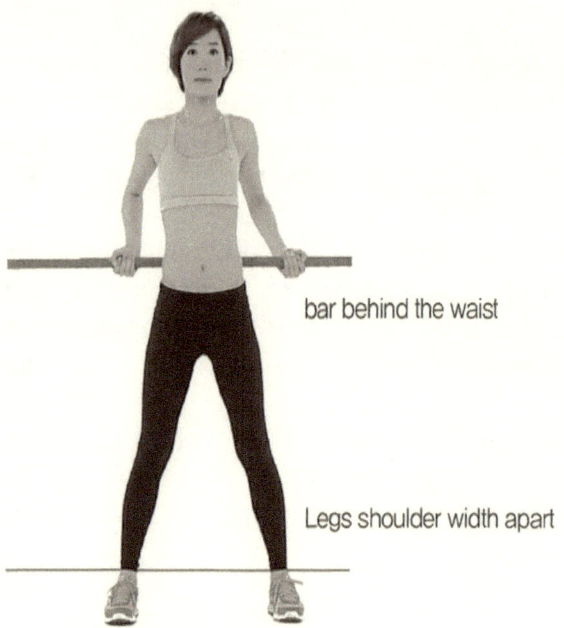

bar behind the waist
Legs shoulder width apart


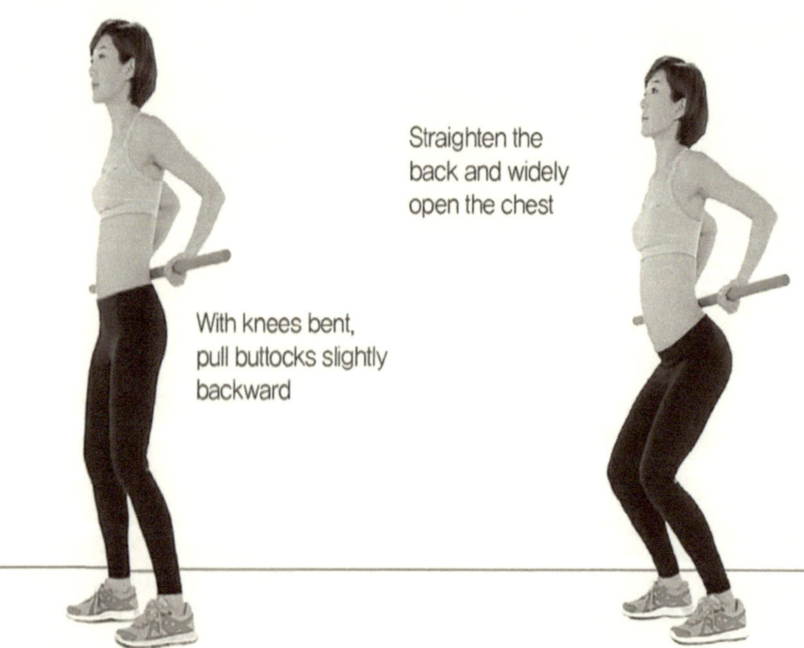

Straighten the
back and widely
open the chest
With knees bent,
pull buttocks slightly
backward

1. Placing the bar behind the waist, hold onto it with both hands as shown and stand with legs shoulder width apart.

2. slightly bend the knees, open the chest, tighten the abdominal muscles and the lower back to prevent the upper body from slouching forward.

3. Bend the knees, straighten the upper body and widely open the chest to make the spine into a C shape while slightly pulling out the buttocks backward.

4. When standing up, do not lock the knees but keep them slightly bent. Bring the buttocks back to the original position while keeping the upper body straight. The reason to not lock the knees is to allow the pelvis to bounce to the rhythm. Repeat the movement #2~4 repetitively.

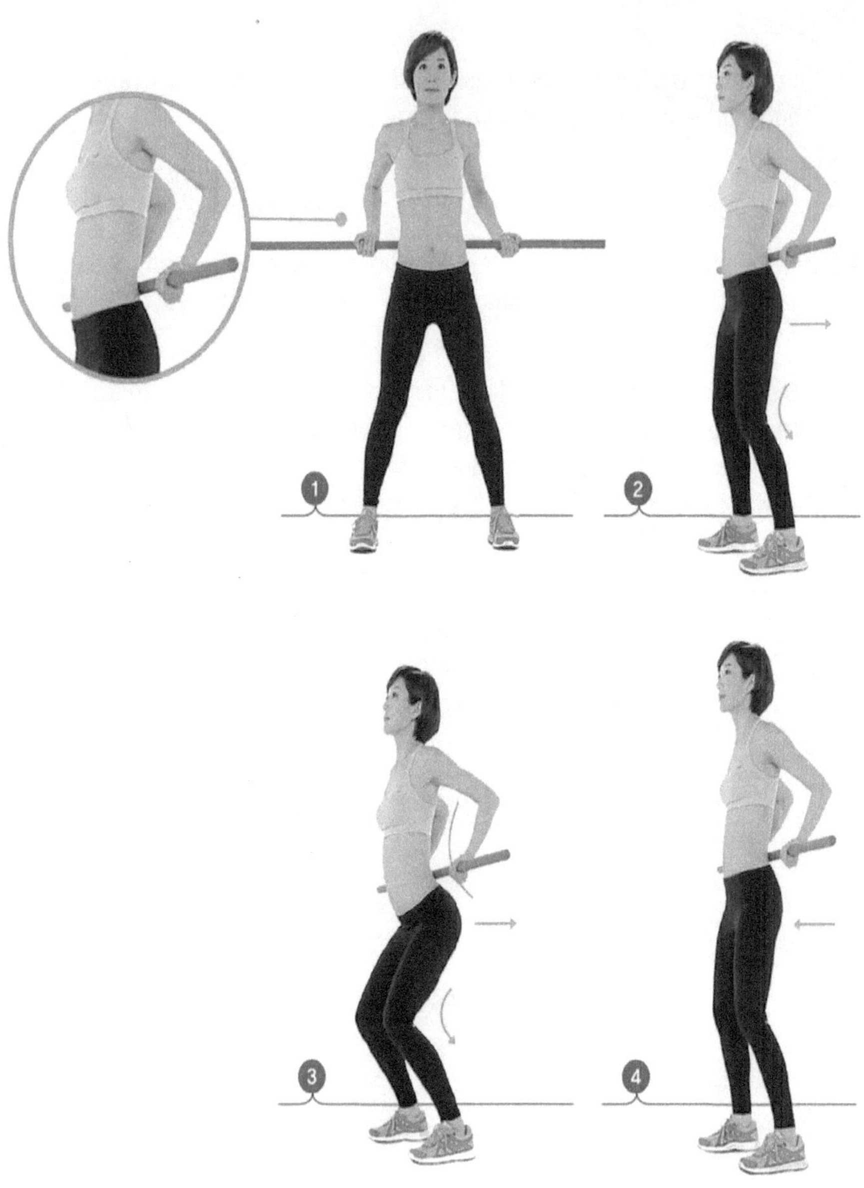





This dance helps the erector spinae muscle and other back muscles to strengthen because you have to maintain an upright posture with the upper body. Placing the bar behind the waist contributes to the development of the pectoralis major muscle because it opens the chest. Also, it helps to build a healthy spinal curve. The neck and the low back become forward curves (c shaped), and the chest and the hips become backward curves (reverse c shaped).

Doing the Electronic Dance steadily helps to keep proper spinal alignment and maintain correct posture. Those who complete the Electronic Dance regularly can increase their upper body muscle mass because the dance has more influence on the spine, the waist and the neck than any other dances.

 Caution

The Electronic Dance can be good for the development of the upper body muscles, but you may cause trauma or pain if you overdo it. Therefore, slowly and precisely follow each movement and do not increase the pace at first. As previously stated, because the Electronic Dance has a huge influence on the upper body, stretch and build up the strength of the muscles through the Down Dance, the Up Dance, and the Techno Dance before you start the Electronic Dance. Patients who have a lack of muscle strength or a disc herniation may have pain, so slow down and gradually increase the pace.

 Example

Mrs. P, an acquaintance of mine, usually stayed away from exercise because of the constant low back pain it caused. This was due to having a weak lower back. She was caught in a vicious cycle of not exercising due to the pain it caused, which in turn made her low back muscles weaker. Having had enough of watching her suffer, I gave her the video clips explaining the Spine Health Dance and told her, "Just trust me on this one and try this whenever you have spare time slowly and gradually."

At first, she was startled and said, "You are telling someone who even hates walking to dance? Will you be responsible for my back if it gets worse and causes pain again?" She ended up taking the video clips as I insisted. When I contacted her about a month later, she replied in a dull voice, "I do it whenever the thought of doing it pops into my head."

It seemed like she was not taking it seriously, so I sincerely asked, "If you thrust me as a doctor, please give it a try". She said OK, but I wondered. 'Would she really dance? She is someone who feels pain and is bedridden by any bit of exercise.'

In about two months, Mrs. P came to me and asked, "Do you have some other kinds of dances? This program is great!" She smiled and gave me a thumbs up. She was skeptical in the beginning but reluctantly tried a couple of times, but the dance was too much for her as she rarely exercised before.

She thought about giving up, but thinking that the person who suggested the dance is not anyone else but her own personal doctor, she followed the movements little by little. With the music on, it was quite addictive and found she could consistently do it even though it was hard.

Because I called her and told her to try it if she really respects me as a doctor, she must have felt pressured to do so. As time passed, she gained some strength and signs of fatigue diminished.

She soon realized that she has not gone to a hospital for over 3 months. In the past, Mrs. P used to visit me three or four times in one month.

Mrs. P said, "The most miraculous thing is that I did not fall down even when I thought I would collapse." She lavished me with her praise and added, "Who would believe that a neurosurgeon tells his patient to dance for pain relief. You are one of a kind."

Although I was flattered by Mrs. P's praise, I was the most excited to hear her say, "I now have the courage to do any kind of exercise and I feel excited to have energy in my everyday life."

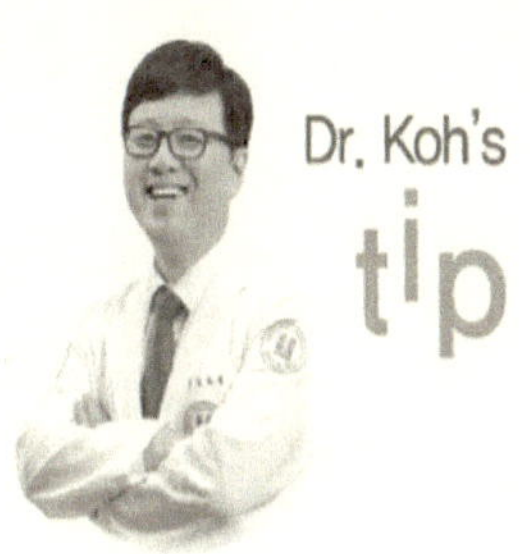


**Pectoralis Major Muscle**

The pectoralis major muscle is a fan shaped muscle located on the chest of the body. The muscle is divided into two regions: the superior region arises from the surface of the sternal area of the clavicle and the inferior region arises from the area of the ribs and the sternum. These muscles end at the intertubercular groove of the humerus. The lateral lip forms the inner wall of the axillary and the muscle inserts on the lateral lip of the intertubercular groove of the humerus.

The pectoralis major muscle has a role that adducts and medially rotates the humerus. The superior region of the muscle flexes the humerus and the inferior region adducts the humerus.

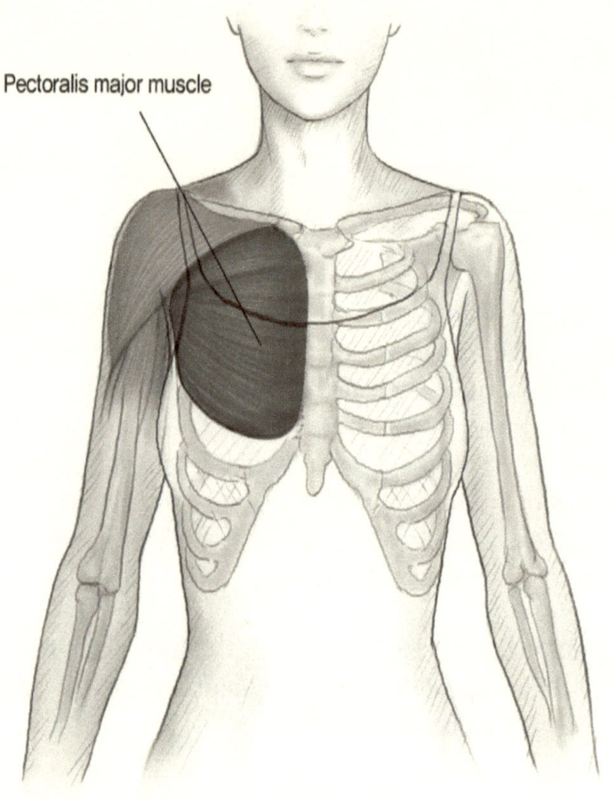

Pectoralis major muscle

# 05
# **ROCKCODE**
# DANCE

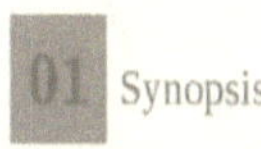 Synopsis

People around the world like to imitate Psy's horse dance from his famous song, Gangnam Style, but they may not know how strong of an effect the dance has. Rockcode Dance is transformed slightly from the horse dance in order to maximize the effects on the body.

The horse dance's movements are moving the buttocks from side to side while stamping the opposite foot. The Rockcode Dance's movements are slightly different by bending the knees a little bit and walking continuously. At this time, the movements are not just walking but bouncing up from the floor as if there are springs under the feet. If you increase the pace, the effects of the dance can be equal to the movements of running.

While walking seems simple and basic at every step, about 200 bones and more than 600 muscles in the body move together and every organ becomes highly active. Walking is simple yet marvelous and scientific.

The Time has published an article titled 'Walk, Don't Run.' The content noted that walking for 30 minutes 5 times a week is the essential requirements for health. These kinds of medical reports have been published through research papers. The World Health Organization recommends walking for 30 minutes daily in order to prevent lifestyle diseases.

There is also a research paper that states walking is very effective for people with high blood pressure. If people walked at a quick pace more than 1 hour a week, their blood pressure went down. This study was done with 207 patients with high blood pressure at the National Institute of Health/Nutrition Research and the National Sanatorium of Central Hospital in Japan.

According to the facts revealed through this research, the effects of walking for an hour at one time versus walking a total of an hour in a week at different times are very similar. The effect was more evident in the group with higher blood pressure.

 Who needs this?

The Rockcode Dance is very good for those who don't exercise or have very little activity. The dance is also effective for people who can no longer find time to exercise. Most of all, the dance is very useful in the middle to older aged adults who have lifestyle disorders since it can have the same effects as walking.

## 03 Basic Movement

Stand with legs shoulder width apart, placing the bar vertical in front of the body. Bending the knees slightly, walk in place, slowly alternating left and right legs. Gradually start stomping the feet, bouncing up from the floor as if there are springs under the feet.

Getting into the rhythm, put the body weight on the bar and walk with the ball of your foot as if you're pecking the floor, using a bouncing motion. After getting used to this movement, you don't need to use the bar anymore. Walking in rhythm, increase the pace as you get better.

Once you're familiar with walking, start hopping, alternating the feet for each step. In the middle of alternating feet, hop twice with the right foot, return to alternating feet, then hop twice with the left foot. Alternately place the ball of the foot closer to the bar while hopping. Then, hop lightly as if you're walking.

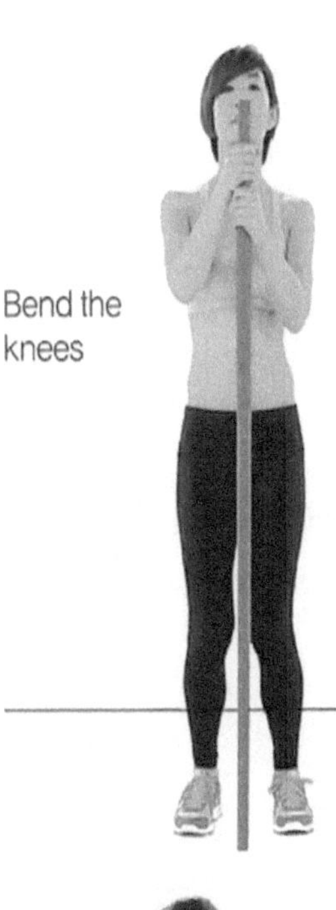

Bend the knees

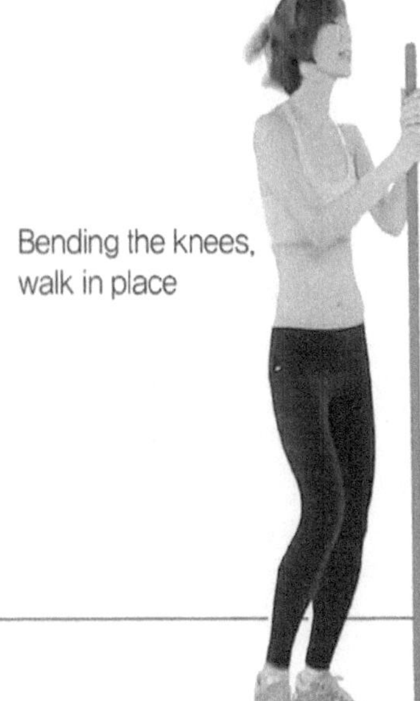

Bending the knees, walk in place

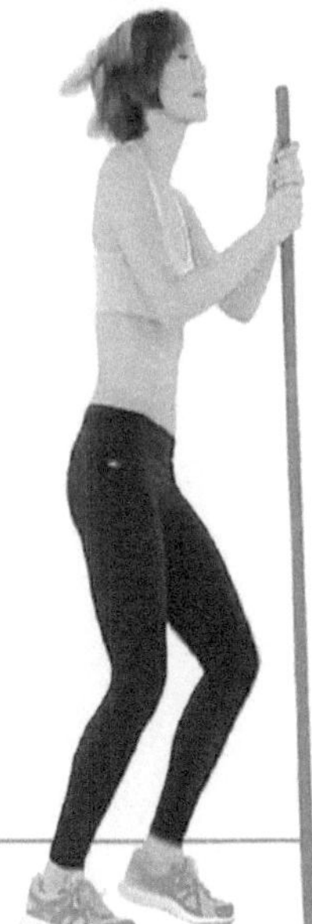

Hop alternately

1 When the dance starts, place the bar vertical in front of the body and hold onto it loosely while standing.

2 Holding onto the bar, bend the knees slightly.

3 Walk while alternately stomping the ball of your foot in the rhythm as if you're riding on a pogo stick. Once you get used to this movement, increase the pace and try walking faster. When you get used to walking, start hopping alternately, twice with the right foot, back to alternating feet, then twice with the left foot. Repeat.

4 When you're familiar with the movement #3, alternately place each foot closer to the bar while hopping. Then slow down the pace by hopping lightly as if you're walking.

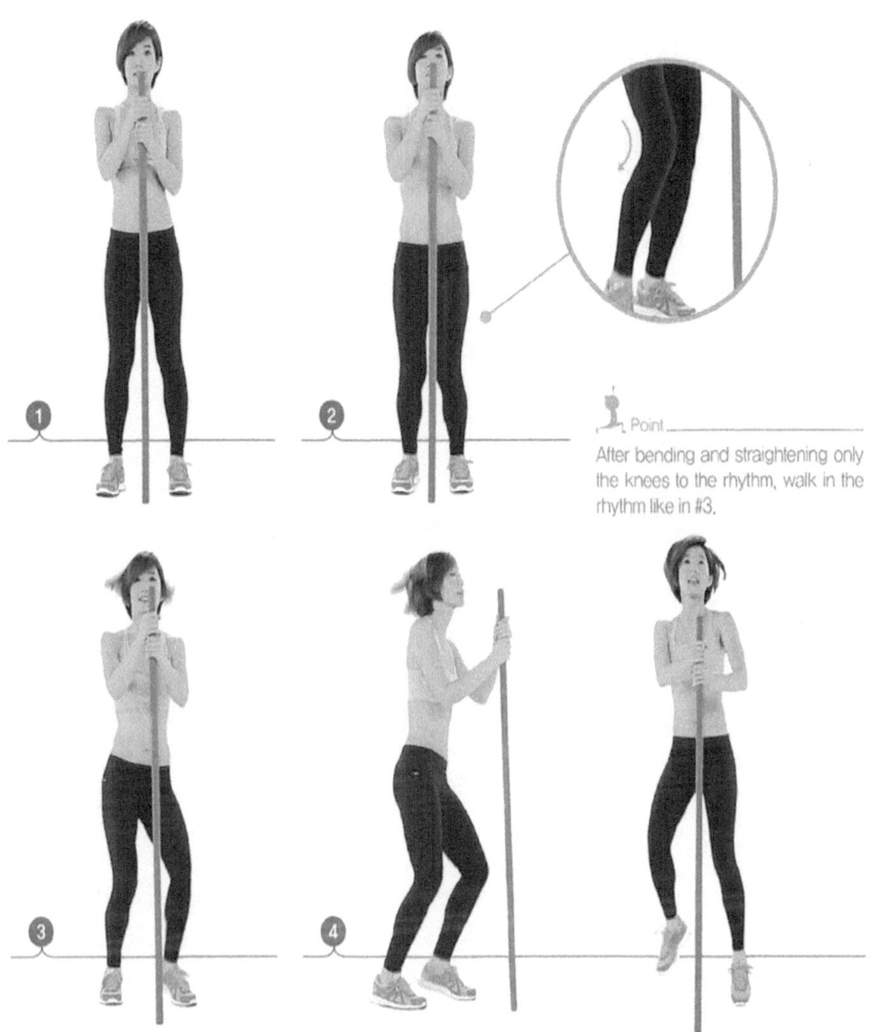



05 Effects

Consistently practicing the Rockcode Dance, which can have the effects of walking and even running, allows patients to strengthen their cardiopulmonary function and improve lifestyle disorders. Thus, it is an effective aerobic exercise for whole body health.

 Caution

I advise you to avoid intense exercise in the beginning, but take time and increase the pace little by little because the Rockcode Dance by itself is more intense than the other dances in this program. If you practice at a high pace, you may experience difficulty breathing.

I recommend older people to increase their duration of exercise gradually, starting from 1~2 minutes each day. If they increase their pace too fast, they may adversely affect their cardiopulmonary function. Those who suffer from severe degenerative knee arthritis should not do this dance.

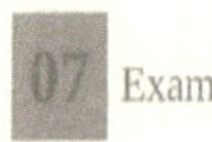 Example

Mr. Y is an entrepreneur in his late 20s. He suffered from low back pain and joint pain because of the constant effect of his obesity on his disc and joints. He is a successful young man who had decided to become an entrepreneur at an early age.

The reason Mr. Y couldn't escape from obesity since middle school was because he couldn't control his eating. He had five meals, each being a full-size meal of an average person in addition to ramen, chicken, and fried foods as snacks.

Due to his obesity, he received warning signals from his body. However, for Mr. Y, the signal for hunger was taken more seriously than the warning signals. Because he couldn't reduce the amount of consumption, there was no chance of resolving the obesity.

Low back pain and joint pain are closely related to obesity. With his body weight much heavier than normal, Mr. Y couldn't get rid of his low back and joint pain. The only way for him to eliminate the pain was by losing weight.

For Mr. Y, managing a diet was the last thing he would do. It was not that he did not exercise at all. He went to the gym after work and walked for two hours. This did not help because after the exercise, he took in more calories than he burned.

Having tried all kinds of popular diet programs and even some supplement pills, Mr. Y failed every time. He was at the point where he had given up on losing weight. When I gave him the video clips of the Down, Up, Techno, Electronic and Rockcode Dance. I explicitly requested that he complete the program at least three to four times a week.

Mr. Y usually visited me about once a month, but this time he came to me within two weeks and complained that his muscles were sore all over. He told me that his body felt so heavy, but he still tried to dance every day as I had suggested.

After providing a simple treatment and prescribing medicine, I encouraged him to continue and to be persistent. Three months later, Mr. Y came to me with a slimmer face. His body was also much slimmer.

Mr. Y smiled and said, "Dr. Koh, other kinds of dances are good too, but the best one for losing weight is the Rockcode Dance. I have used a treadmill for a while, but my body wasn't as responsive to it like the dance. Excited with the changes brought by the dance, I have replaced snacks with water or tea. It might not be apparent, but I have lost 9kg so far."

Mr. Y has lost weight up to the point where he is no longer obese. From time to time, he feels pain in the knees and ankles, hopping too much on the pogo stick, but it is just a result of excessive exercise, and not a serious problem.

Mr. Y can now exercise for a longer time not only because of losing weight but also because his movements feel noticeably lighter. He used to get short of breath when he moved more than usual, but after starting the dance, he is gradually overcoming that issue.

Because Mr. Y got good results from the dance, all his family members became fanatics about the Spine Health Dance. Both his parents, suffer from diabetes and high blood pressure and are hoping that dancing every day will make things better. His sister, who has no health problems, is also dancing the Spine Health Dance just to shape her body.

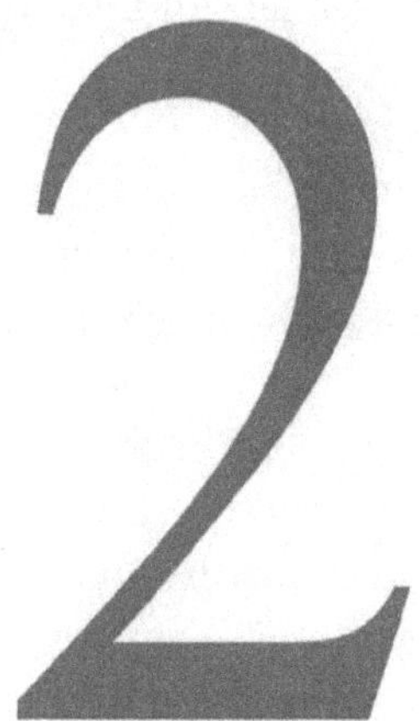

# 2

Spine Health Dance Therapy

## Gym Ball
## Dance

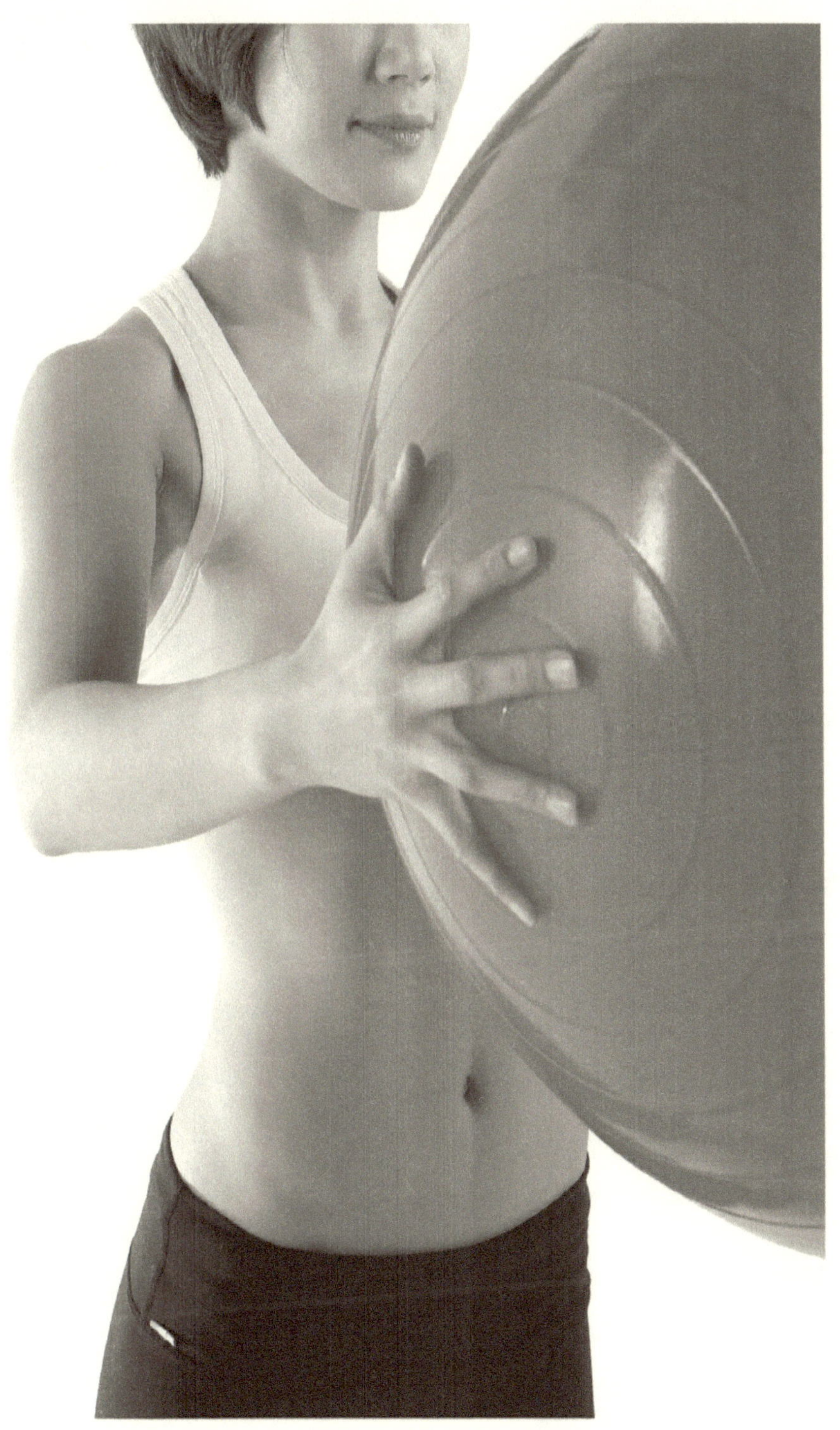

Why do I ask you to use a gym ball with the dance? There are several reasons. First of all, as I stated earlier you can solve the problem of when you feel awkward dancing with bare hands, and most of all, dancing with a gym ball is great for your arms and shoulders.

Also, you can focus on the leg movements when you have a gym ball in your hands. Furthermore, the middle aged and older adults may feel psychological comfort with exercises when they hold a gym ball instead of their bare hands. A gym ball can also be used as a chair when you rest during the exercise.

I would like to omit the reference about 'who needs this,' 'the effects,' and 'the caution' in the Gym Ball Dance because they are similar to those of the Stretching Bar Dance.

# 01
# **DOWN**
# DANCE

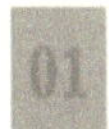 Synopsis

Down Dance is like the first dance when people learn to dance at a club. Both the Gym Ball Down Dance and the Bar Down Dance have same effects. However, people with a weak abdomen can extend the upper body easily if they push a gym ball to the stomach slightly.

 Who needs this?

The Gym Ball Down Dance is basically a full body workout. At first, the lower body muscles such as the quadriceps femoris muscle and the hamstring muscle are strengthened while bending and straightening the knees. The abdominal muscles are strengthened while extending and bending the upper body. Also, the neck and the waist get stronger because the erector spinae muscle is strengthened.

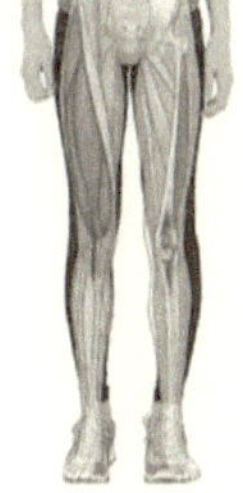 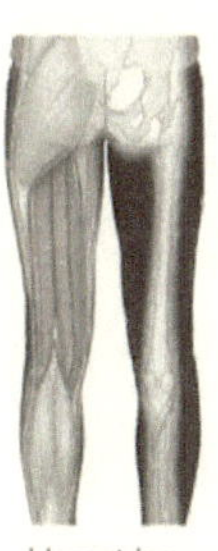 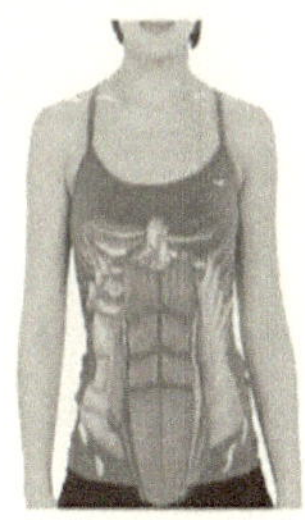 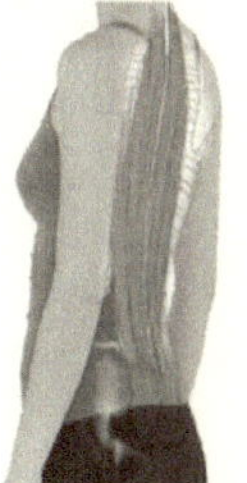

| Quadriceps femoris muscle | Hamstring muscle | Abdominal muscles | Erector spinae muscle |

 Basic Movement

In the standing position with the back straight and legs shoulder width apart, hold a gym ball naturally up to the height of the belly. Bending the knees and holding the core tight, slightly lean the upper body backward. Straightening the knees, raise up the upper body. It is important to keep the core tight to prevent the body from swaying. Slightly pushing the belly with the gym ball helps to tighten the abdomen.

Once you get used to this movement, try mixing with another movement, bending and straightening the knees while lifting the gym ball above the head. Repeat these two movements 4 times each.

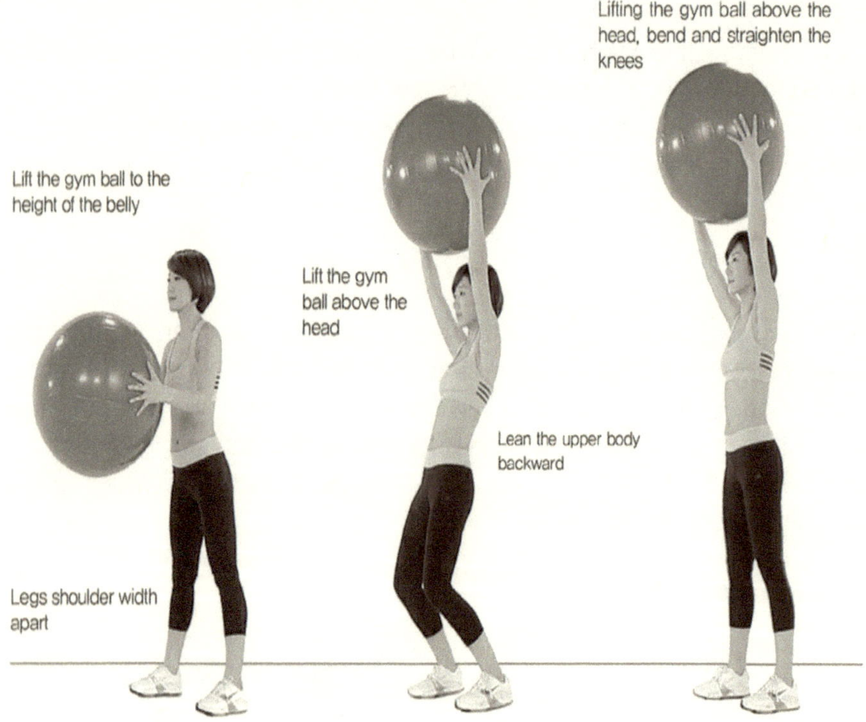


**04** Details

**1** Stand with the legs shoulder width apart while keeping the back straight, hold a gym ball to the height of the belly.

**2** Bend the knees and slightly lean the upper body backward, tightening the core and keeping the upper body straight to prevent the buttocks from falling back.

**3** Straightening the knees, raise up the upper body and stand upright. Repeat the movement #1~3 at least 4 times.

**4** After repeating #1~3 4 times, bend the knees in the same way as the above and this time strongly raise the gym ball above the head. Maintain the upper body straight, do not lean backwards.

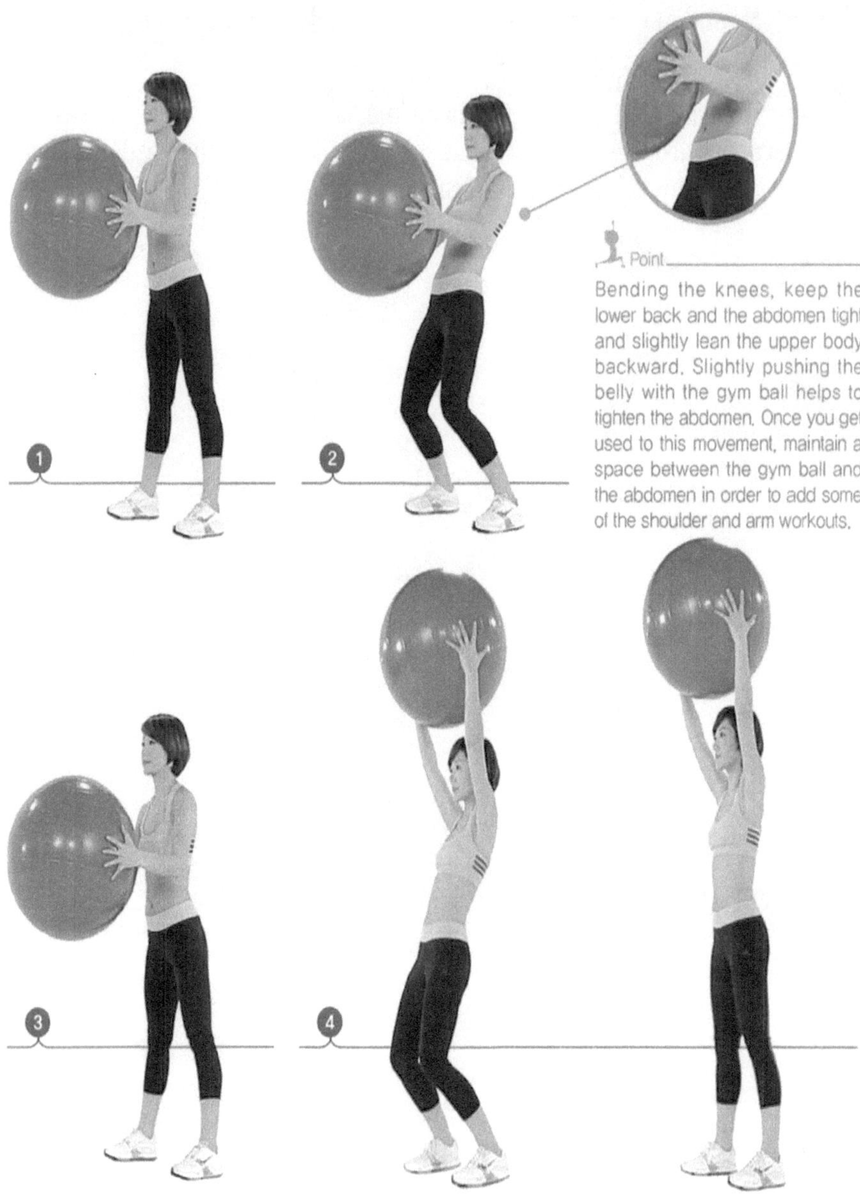



Bending the knees, keep the lower back and the abdomen tight and slightly lean the upper body backward. Slightly pushing the belly with the gym ball helps to tighten the abdomen. Once you get used to this movement, maintain a space between the gym ball and the abdomen in order to add some of the shoulder and arm workouts.

# 02
# **UP**
# DANCE



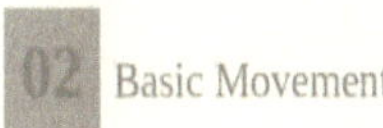

The Gym Ball Up Dance is an intensive full body workout, so start slowly at first and increase the pace slowly as the workout gets easier. Then you can apply other movements such as raising the arms with the gym ball over head.

## 02 Basic Movement

With the back straight, bend the knees and hold a gym ball at a natural position as if you are gently hugging the ball. Straightening the knees and rising up, slightly lean the upper body forward while keeping the legs and the core tight. The effectiveness of this exercise is maximized when the core and the legs are tightened to prevent the buttocks from falling back because it helps to stimulate the muscles in the upper body.

Keep the upper body straight when bending the knees, lift one leg and lean the upper body forward before straightening the knees. Alternate legs and repeat this movement twice.

Then walk in place 8 times, holding the gym ball naturally. When walking in place, bring up one knee towards the chest and slightly bend the other leg on the ground.

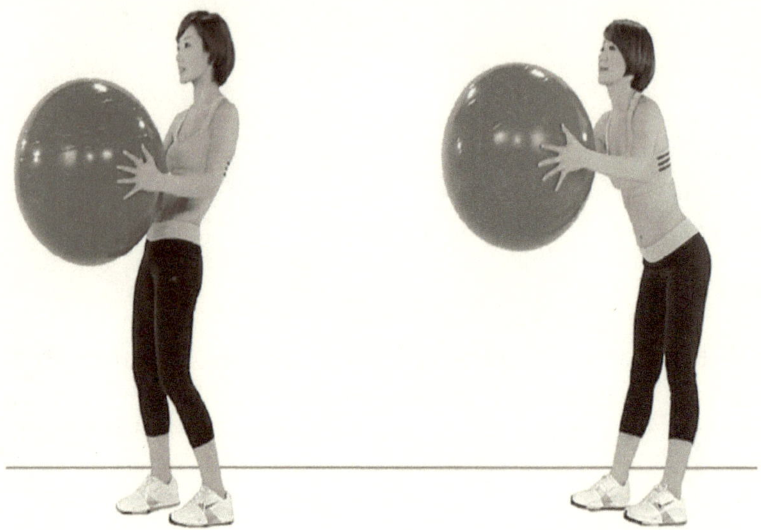

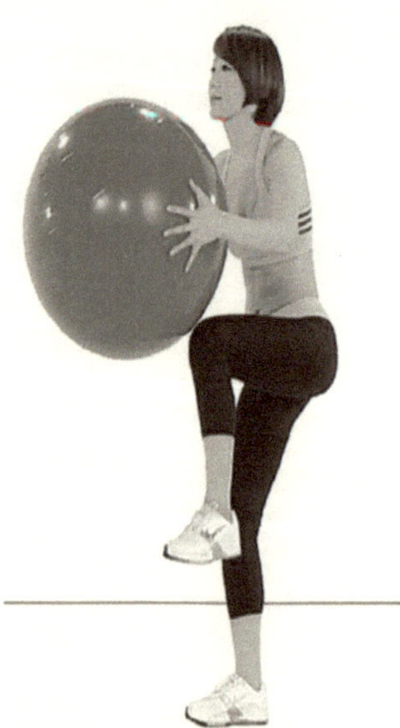

**1** Bend the knees slightly to 45~55 degrees and get into position, naturally holding a gym ball. Straighten the upper body and tighten the core to prevent the buttocks from falling back.

**2** Strongly push the ground and straighten the knees as you shout out "One" while leaning the upper body slightly forward. When leaning forward, tighten the entire upper body to make the movement lively.

**3** Lift one leg as you straighten the bent knees to stand up straight. Keep holding onto the gym ball naturally.

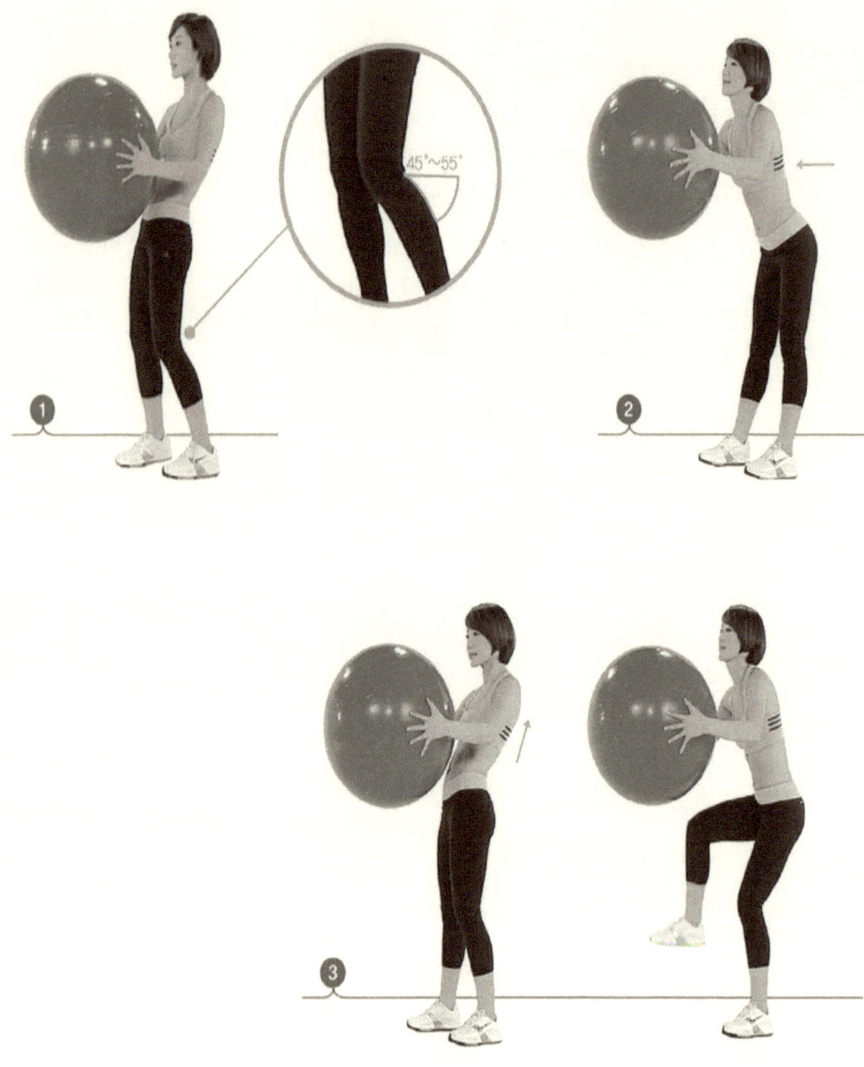


4 As you bring the leg back to the ground, try not to let the buttocks fall back as you did in step 2 and slightly lean the upper body forward.

5 As you bend and straighten the knees again, lift the other leg as if pushing it slightly outward. Repeat the movement #1~5 twice.

6 Holding the gym ball in the same position, walk in place, bringing one knee towards the chest and slightly bending the other knee. The exercise

is more effective if the knees touch the gym ball softly, making the ball
bounce as you walk.

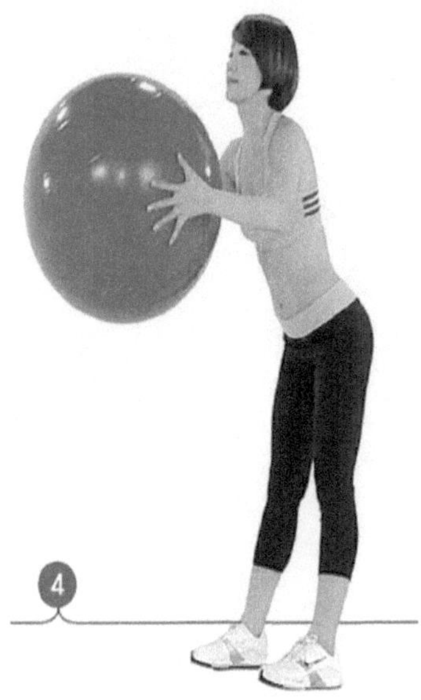

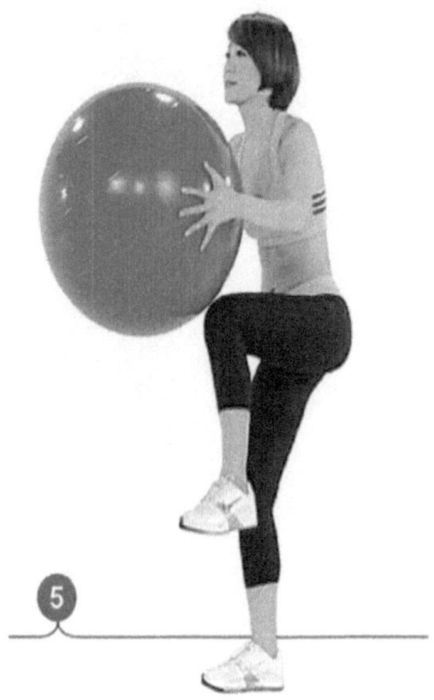

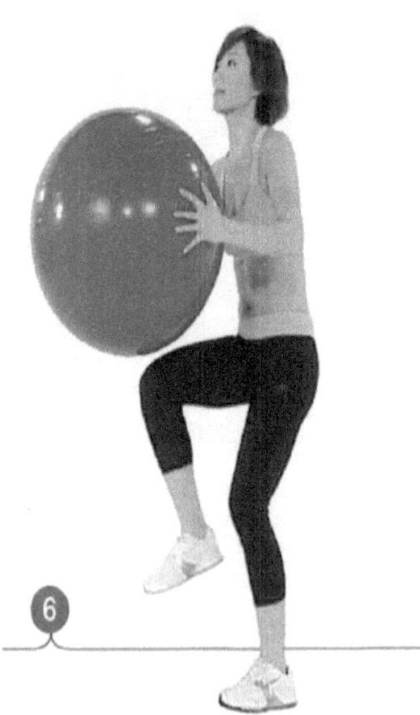

# 03
# TECHNO
## DANCE

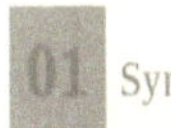 Synopsis

The Techno Dance which uses the rotation of the waist and the movement of the pelvis is a full body workout to strengthen hip muscles as well as the upper body. Because the dance has a higher physical demand on the body, those who have a disc problem or sciatic neuralgia should consult a physician before completing this dance.

## 02 Basic Movement

Holding a gym ball at the chest with pelvis pushed slightly forward, push the pelvis to the left and right alternately. When moving the pelvis, make sure the knees are not bent. Since the gym ball is bigger than the bar, it prevents the upper body from slouching and the center of gravity from shifting backward and makes it easy to tighten the core.

After swaying the pelvis left and right twice, strongly twist the upper body to face the moving direction of the pelvis. When adding rotational force to the upper body, it is important to make it quick and strong.

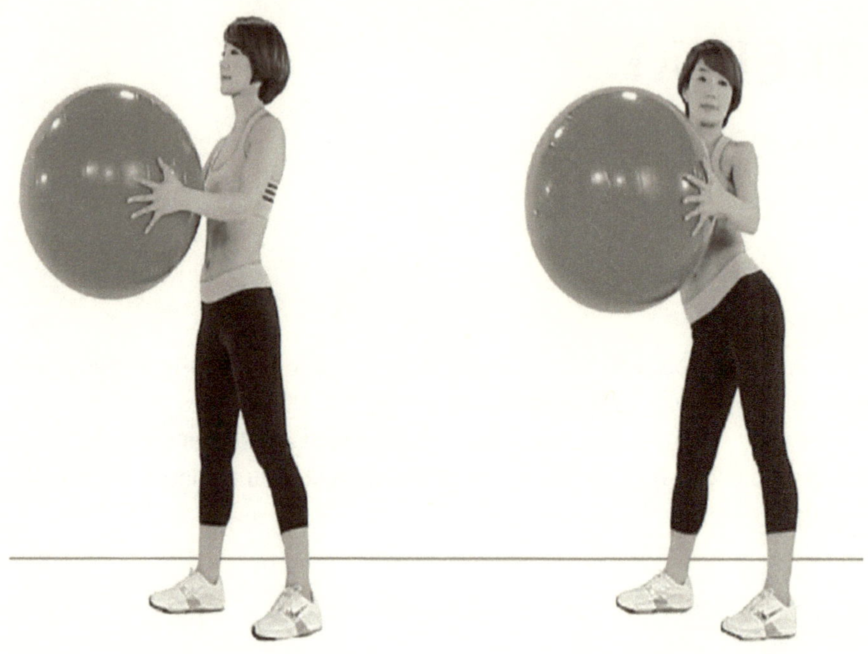

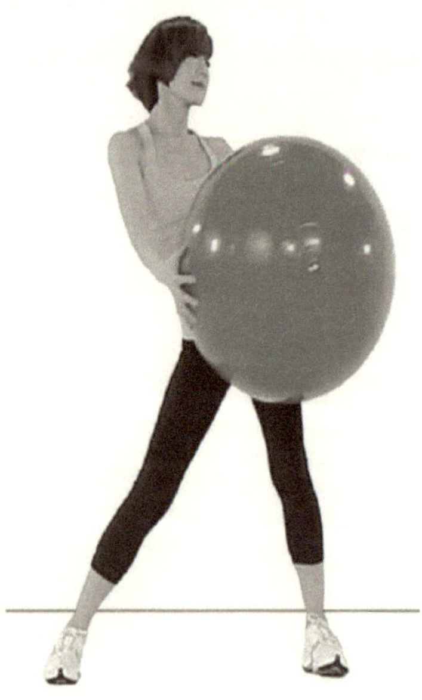

**1** Stand with the legs shoulder width apart and lift a gym ball up to the chest.

**2** Tightening the core to prevent the buttocks from falling back, shift the center of gravity of the upper body slightly backward.

**3** In posture #2, lightly sway the pelvis left and right twice. Then, strongly twist the upper body to face the moving direction of the pelvis. Turn the head at the same time.

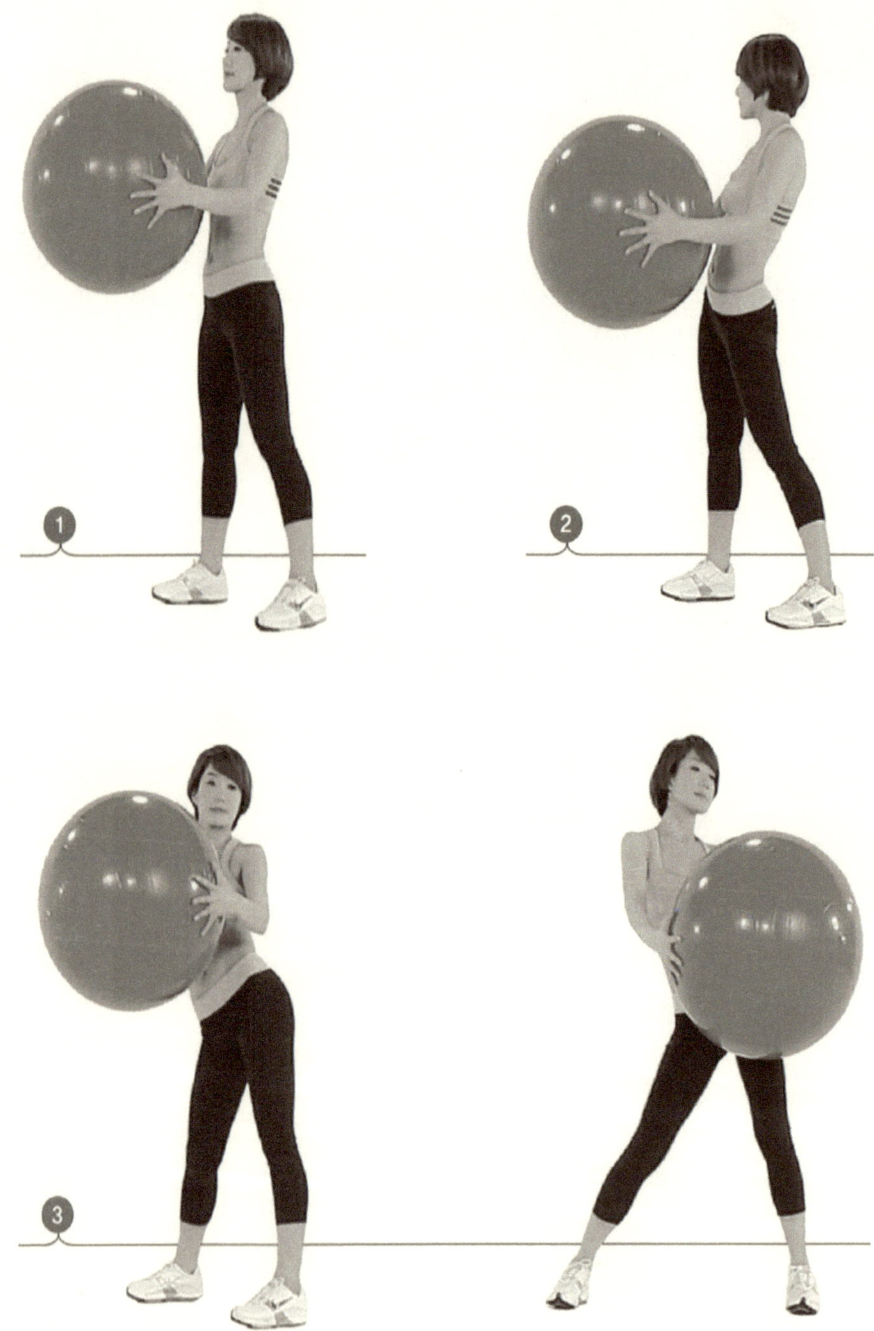

**4** Lift the gym ball above the head and sway the pelvis left and right. Strongly twist the upper body to face the moving direction of the pelvis and turn the head too.

⚠ For those whose legs go numb or buttocks get unevenly weighted after sitting for a long time, keep the rotating angle small when twisting the upper body to prevent overloading the disc.

⚠ For those 50s and older who may have lost the full capability of their vestibular organs, keep head and eyes facing front or turn the head just slightly and twist the upper body with the waist to prevent dizziness.

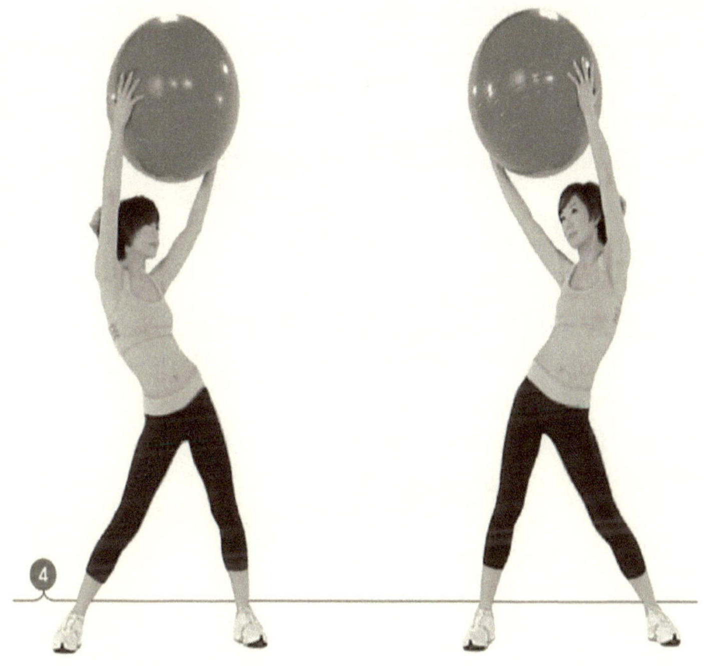

# 04

# ELECTRONIC
## DANCE

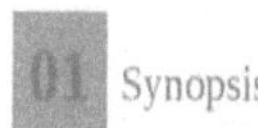 Synopsis

In the Bar Electronic Dance, holding the bar behind the back naturally helped to keep the upper body upright while pulling out the buttocks backward. However, in the Gym Ball Electronic Dance, your upper body may become slightly bent and the center of gravity may shift forward because of the gym ball weight. Therefore, you have to focus on keeping the upper body upright.

## 02 Basic Movement

Hold a gym ball naturally and stand with legs shoulder width apart. Bend and straighten the knees, but do not lock them keeping them slightly bent so that it's easier to bounce to the rhythm.

When bending the knees, open the chest and slightly pull out the buttocks backward while keeping the upper body upright. Do not pull out the buttocks backward too much or too little and keep the abdomen tight. Gradually get into the rhythm and repeat the same movement.

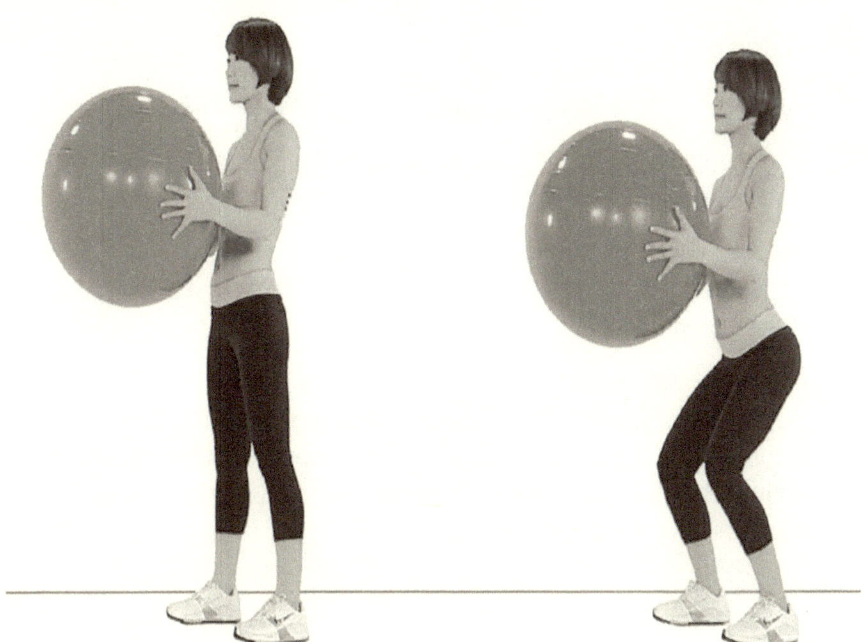

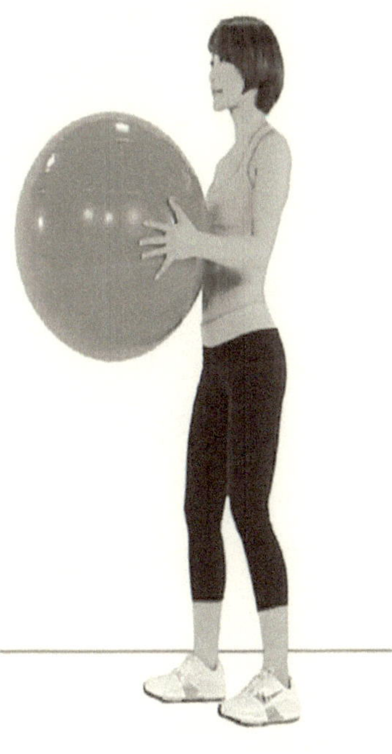

1. Hold a gym ball naturally and stand with legs shoulder width apart.

2. Bend the knees, open the chest and tighten the core to prevent the upper body from leaning forward.

3. Bending the knees, slightly pull out the buttocks backward while straightening the upper body and opening the chest to make a 'C' shape with your spine.

4. When you are standing up, keep the knees slightly bent rather than locking them. Then push the buttocks back to the original position while keeping the upper body upright. The reason for keeping the knees slightly bent is to make it easy to bounce the pelvis to the rhythm. Repeat the movement #2~4 continuously.

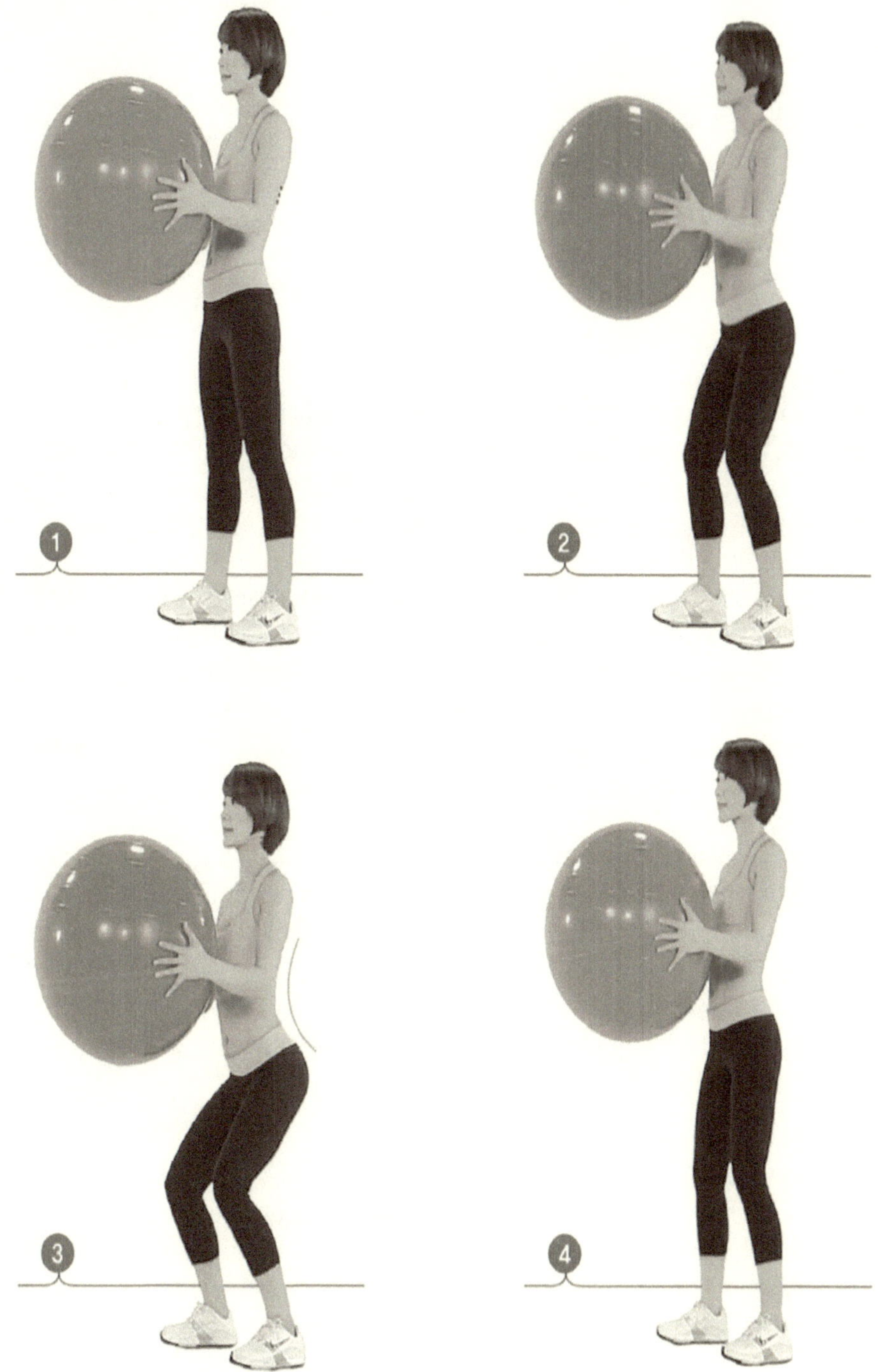

# 05
# ROCKCODE
## DANCE



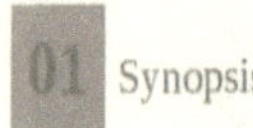 Synopsis

As introduced earlier, the Bar Rockcode Dance is hard to keep the balance of the body because you have to exercise with the knees slightly bent. That is why a bar is used as a support tool to keep your balance. Using a gym ball for this exercise maximizes the effects as there is no longer a support tool.

Walking and running which are typical aerobic exercises have great effects on the body. People can walk slowly with the Rockcode Dance, but if they get into the rhythm and try walking faster with the hops, they will have both walking and running effects. Doing the Rockcode Dance for 10 minutes may have the same effect as walking for 30 minutes. Also, the Rockcode Dance can be more effective than treadmill workout.

For the patients who have a tilted right pelvis and an outward facing right leg, the titled pelvis may get realigned (if the dance is performed with the right leg rotated in). If they have a tilted left pelvis, rotate the left leg inward and do the dance. In this case, if performed for a long time, the pelvic problem may be over corrected, so they should not exceed 1 minute. Also, they have to dance with the legs positioned normally after the alignment of the pelvis.

02 Basic Movement

Stand with the legs shoulder width apart and hold a gym ball naturally. Bend the knees slightly and slowly walk, alternating the left and right foot. As you start walking, use the rebounding force at the feet and walk as if you are lightly hopping. When you get used to this movement, you may increase the pace.

When the hopping walk gets familiar, try hopping with the right foot twice in the middle of hopping alternately, bring it back to alternate hopping, then hop with the left foot twice. Repeat. In addition, you can cross over each foot alternately inward as you hop and then return to the hopping walk.

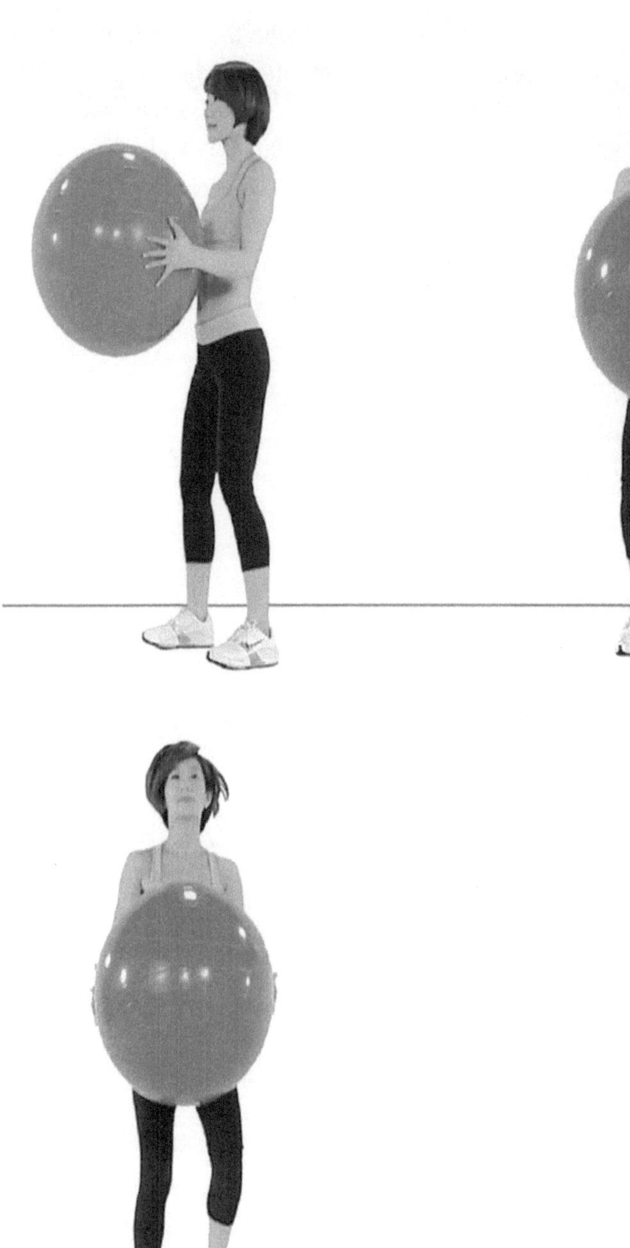

1 Hold a gym ball naturally and stand with the legs shoulder width apart.

2 Bend the knees moderately.

3 With knees kept slightly bent, walk slowly alternating left and right foot.

4 Alternating each foot, walk in the rhythm as if you are riding on a pogostick. When you get familiar with this movement, increase the pace and try walking faster. After getting used to walking, try hopping alternating feet, hop twice with the right foot, alternate again, then hop twice with the left foot.

5 Once #4 gets familiar, hop while crossing over each foot alternately inward. Then slow down the pace by hopping lightly as if you are walking.

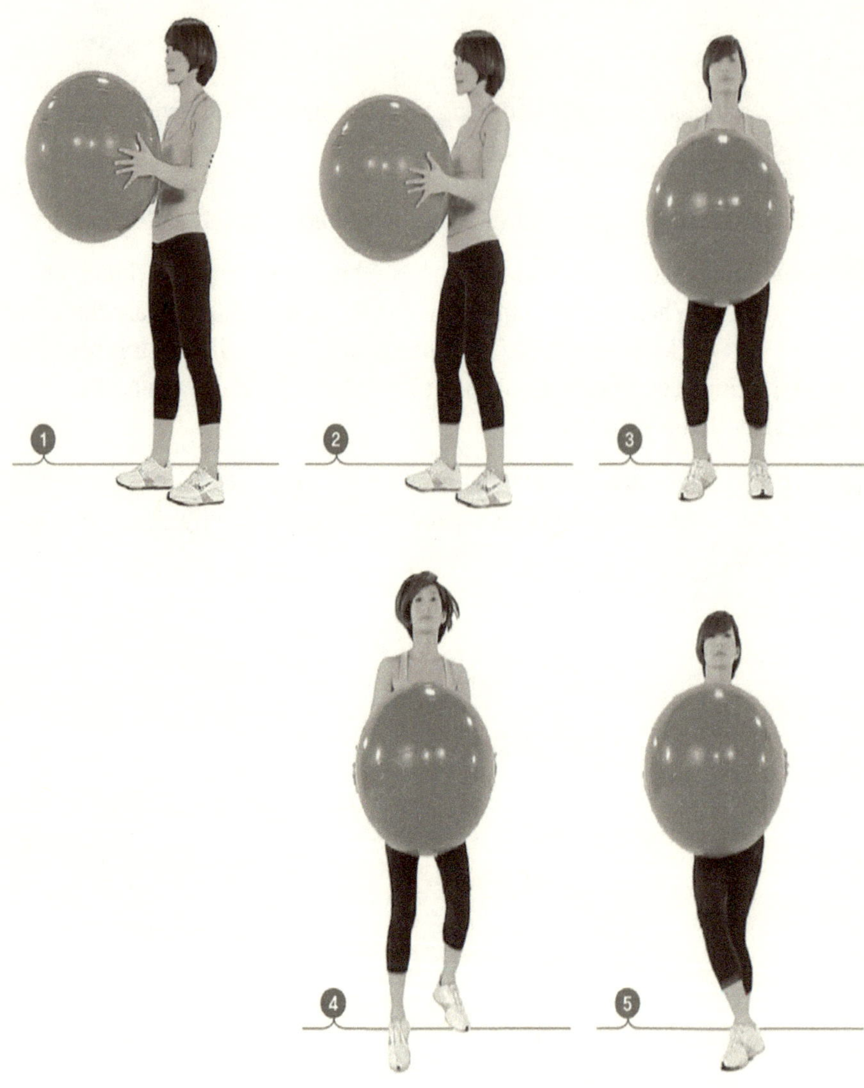

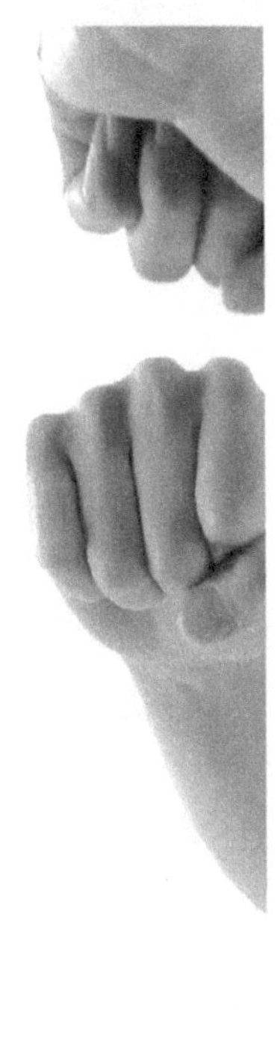

# 3



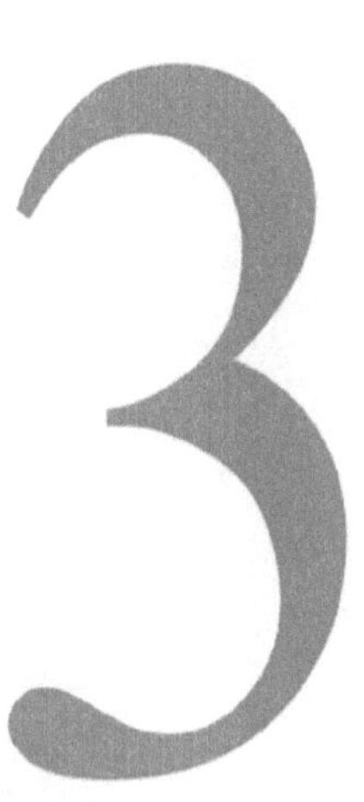

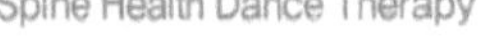

# Dance
# for Body
# Alignment

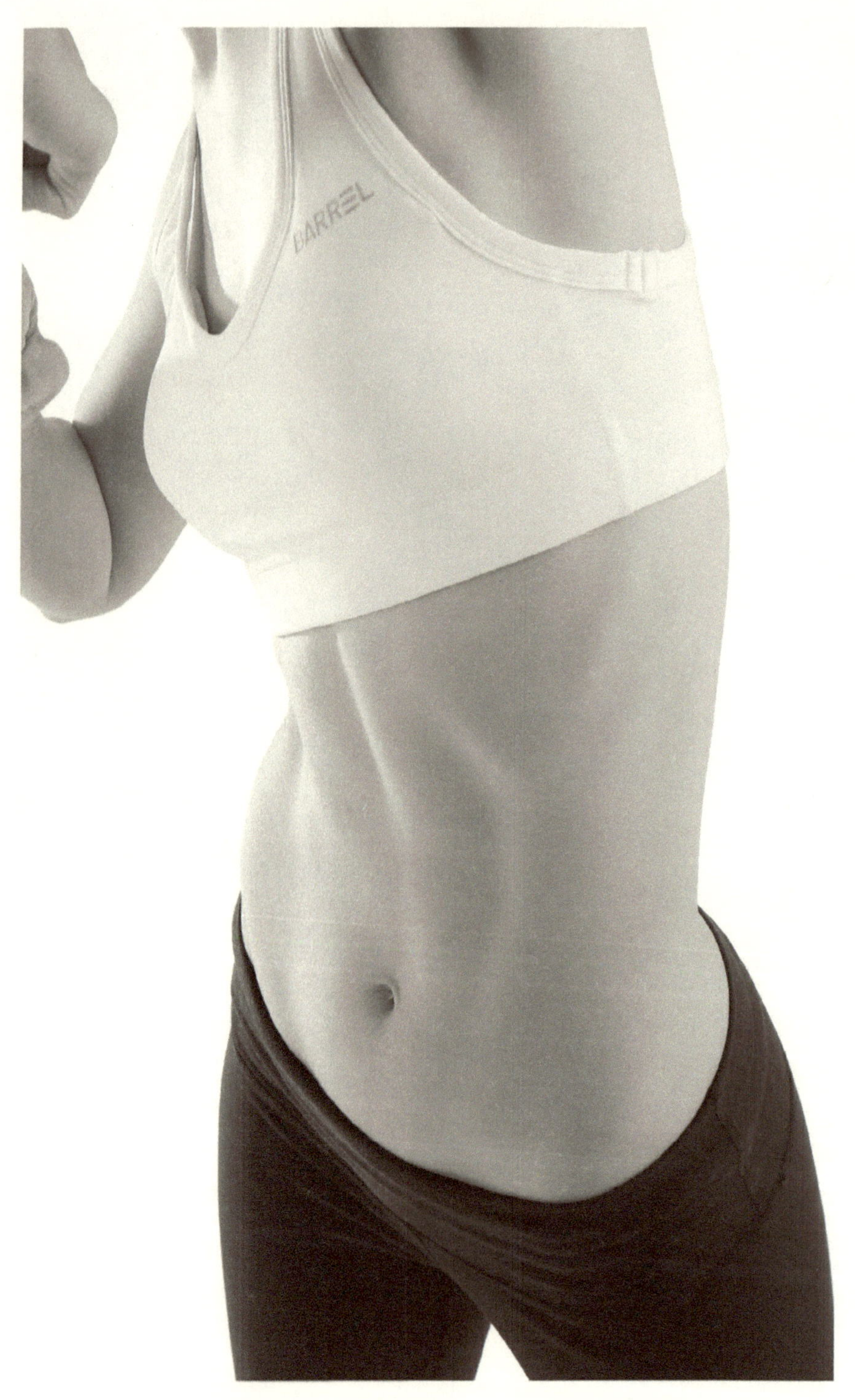
BARREL

The reason why the pelvis can be tilted or a body type gets altered is that the bones are twisted from their original locations due to bad habits, work environment, lifestyle, or unexpected or unnoticeable micro traumas. Serious stress may also lead to a change in body shape.

as such, skeletal changes make growing muscles unevenly positioned and eventually cause asymmetric conditions. If these conditions persist, nerves and blood vessels in the imbalanced muscles are compromised and even worse, they may develop a serious problem such as sensation changes and pain.

If a crooked spine presses on the central nervous system, its related organs are influenced. This mechanism is an established fact through eastern and western medicine. Therefore, we shouldn't ignore the asymmetric changes that occur in the body because the changes will eventually become a problem even if they are unnoticeable now.

# 01

# PELVIC
# ALIGNMENT
# DANCE

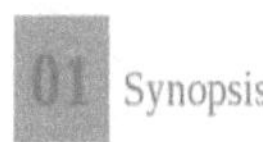 Synopsis

Body misalignment, especially in the pelvis, is very common. Only one in a thousand people is completely normal. Those who have pelvic misalignment find that their pants or skirts go back to one side when they wear them, their underwear is wedged between the buttocks due to the twisting, or their trouser cuffs are worn down on one side due to the difference of the right and left pelvic heights. Shoes can also be worn down more at one heel and fall apart easily because of the imbalance of weight on both legs.

If patients have a lumbar spinal misalignment with an asymmetric pelvis, sometimes their navel is not centered. In this case, this can develop an imbalance of the whole body, causing chronic fatigue and abnormalities. If patients ignore the situation, some serious conditions such as scoliosis or kyphosis could develop.

The biggest reason for the pelvic misalignment is repeated bad habits, such as uneven sitting or standing for long periods of time, sitting with the legs crossed, or sleeping only on the side. Unexpected trauma or accidents can also cause the pelvic misalignment.

When men carry a wallet in their back pocket and sit in a chair or in the car, one side of the pelvis is pushed by the wallet's thickness and as the wallet pushes the buttock, the front of the pelvis drops. If this position is maintained over time, the spine will also misalign.

If you leave a pelvic misalignment as it is, it may lead to the spinal misalignment, which then presses on the central nervous system and can cause problems with muscles, joints and organs. In this case, low back pain and shoulder discomfort may also follow. Furthermore, poor circulation, neuro-transmission system abnormality, hormonogenesis and hormone-transmission abnormality, and so on can also appear. The misalignment can also lead to irregular menstruation, menstrual pain, fertility problems, sexual dysfunction, and more.

The Pelvic Alignment Dance can help a tilted pelvis back to normal within a minute. At first, you have to know which side the pelvis is misaligned before doing the dance.

The easiest way to self-examine is closing your eyes and walking in place for 40 steps. The sense of vision helps us determine the direction when your eyes are open. However, when you close your eyes and march in place, your brain will guide you to step in the right direction through the proprioceptive input which contribute to the sense of position of self and movement. If your pelvis is tilted, you will walk in place towards the direction where your pelvis is misaligned.

If the right side of the pelvis is misaligned, the body will turn to the right. On the other hand, if the left side of the pelvis is misaligned, the body will turn to the left. When the body turns to the right, internally rotate the right leg and place the left leg in the normal position. Then stand firmly to prevent the lower body from moving freely and sway the pelvis left and right for a minute.

You have to move the sacroiliac joints in order to align the pelvis in the proper position, so twist the upper body in the direction of the pelvic movement.

For the opposite case, do it in the same way on the misaligned side of the pelvis. I advise you to exercise for one minute 2~3 times a day and do it regularly for more than 3 months.

An important part of the dance is that you dance for a minute and that your legs must not move. Naturally place the arms at your side during the dance or move them back a little bit if you want to make the exercise more effective.

As explained earlier, the Pelvic Alignment Dance is for those who have pelvic misalignment after inspecting their own pelvis. However, if people don't have any problem with their pelvis and want to make all the muscles of the body, especially the side muscles, strengthened, place both legs in the normal position symmetrically and do the dance.

## 03 Basic Movement

Stand with feet pointing forward and shoulder width apart, then turn the foot on the misaligned side of the pelvis towards the middle. Stand firmly to prevent the lower body from moving freely, then sway the pelvis left and right. To move the sacroiliac joints to align the pelvis in the proper position, twist the upper body in the direction of the pelvic movement.
Dance for less than a minute, close the eyes and walk in place for 40 steps.
If the pelvis is aligned back to normal, place both legs in the normal position and do the same dance again. If the pelvis is not yet aligned, go through the aligning process for a minute again, check if it worked, then do the dance.

Turn the foot on the misaligned side of the
pelvis towards the middle

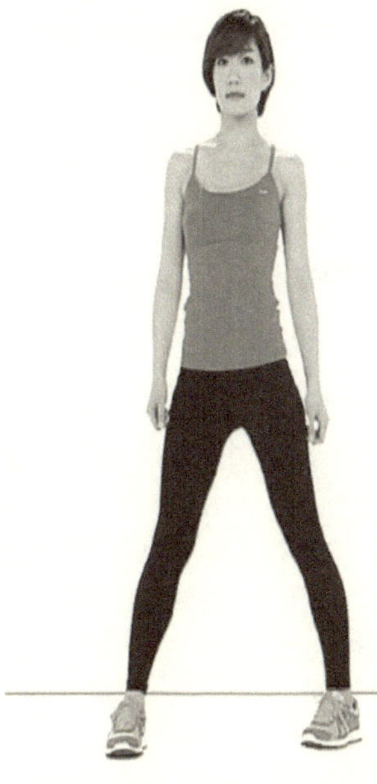

For the case where left side of
the pelvis is misaligned

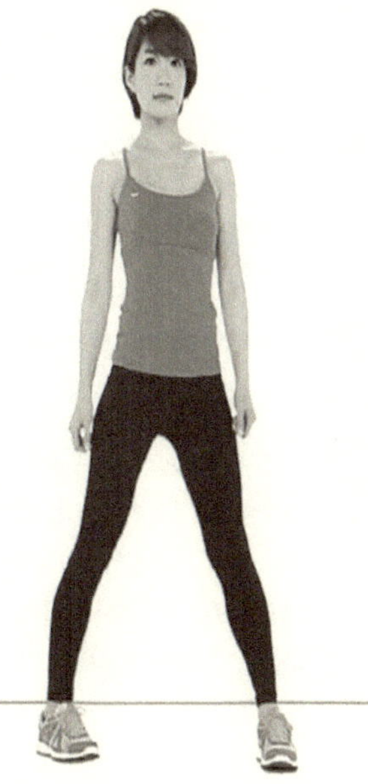

For the case where right side
of the pelvis is misaligned

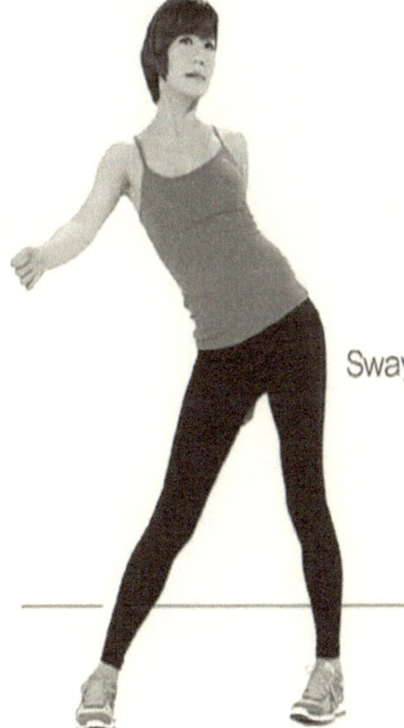

Sway the pelvis left and right

1. To self-examine on which side the pelvis is misaligned, close the eyes and walk in place for 40 steps.

2. The body will turn in the direction of the pelvic misalignment.

3. Turn the foot on the misaligned side of the pelvis inward and hold the lower body tight to prevent it from moving freely.

4. Slightly bring the arms backward, hold the core tight, and sway the pelvis left and right twice.

5. In the position #4, strongly twist the upper body in the direction of the pelvic movement. The legs must not move. Repeat dancing as explained for a minute and self-examining as in #1. When the pelvis is facing forward, spread the feet normally and continue the dance, twisting the upper body in the direction of the pelvic movement.

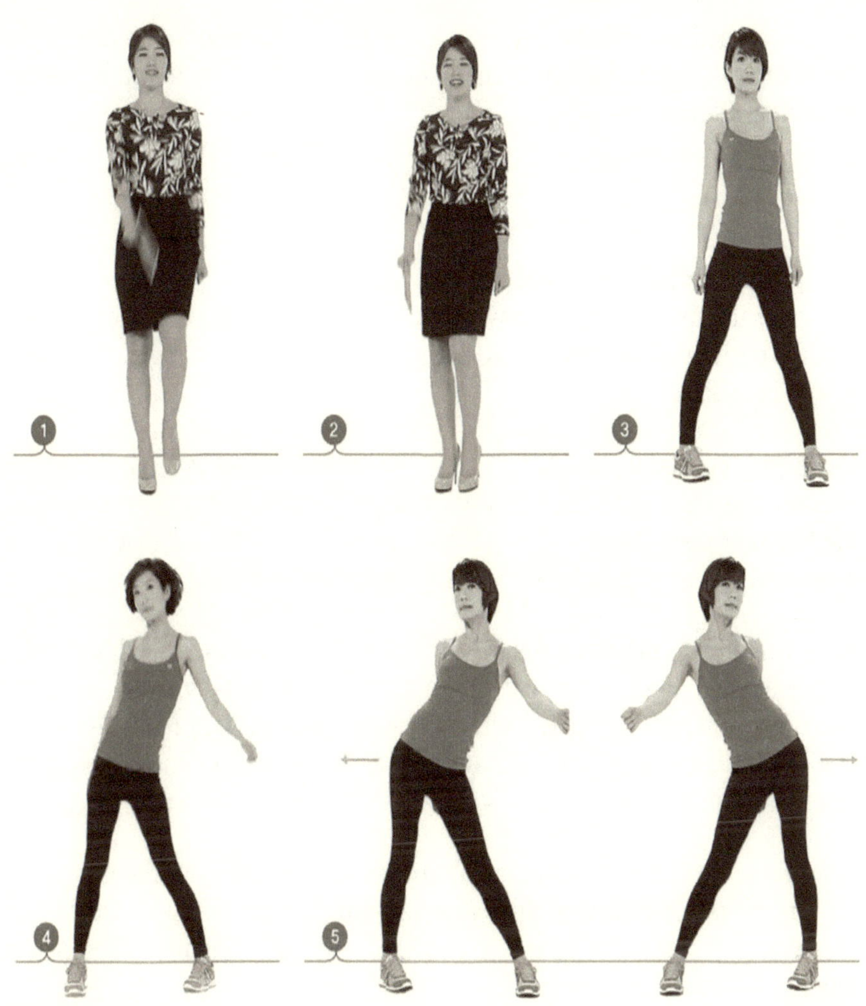



## 05 Effects

The greatest effect of the dance is the correction of pelvic misalignment. When you rotate the upper body, the sacroiliac joints and the side muscles are strengthened. When you hold the lower body tight to prevent it from moving freely, the waist and the lower body muscles such as gluteus medius, gluteus maximus are strengthened.

## 06 Caution

Do not exceed one minute. If you do, the pelvis will be over corrected. An over corrected pelvis falls back into place in about 3 hours, if you happen to exceed one minute.

 **Example**

Ms. L who works as a model came to me with a face of concern. When I asked for the reason, she confessed that it was because her designer told her that the position of her pelvis has changed when she was fitting clothes prior to a fashion show.

She hadn't noticed before, but recently she sees that there is a big difference between the heights of left and right side of her pelvis. Ms. L was worried that she may need surgery. The result of the diagnosis showed that it was not a serious case, but the right side of her pelvis was misaligned.

After listening to the diagnosis, Ms. L was relieved and expressed her desire to get aligned right away and return to the stage. I taught her the self-examining methods and pelvis aligning dance movements. I reminded to her that it will align the pelvis right away, but it needs to be done consistently; otherwise it may return to the misaligned position.

After some time, Ms. L called me in excitement and said, "I like how I can realign my pelvis in a way that is neither difficult nor boring. I taught this dance to my friends around me and they are busy aligning their pelvis through self-examining methods."

Ms. S, a university student, was checking her body one day and was surprised to find out that her pelvis location is different from normal and she came to see me.

She noticed for a while that one side of her shoes wore out faster than the other, but she didn't care that much about it. However, recently, she noticed that the waist line of her pants or skirts tilted to one side.

Ms. S asked in frustration, "If the pelvis is tilted this much, wouldn't it make giving birth more difficult?" It is true that if the pelvic misalignment is left untreated, it could end up in a more serious malposition.

I taught her the dance movements for pelvic realignment, as well as the self-examining methods. Ms. S seemed quite surprised at the treatment methods. Although she seemed mistrusting, I insisted that she consistently exercise the dance program 2 to 3 times a day for over 3 months.

When Ms. S visited me after a few months, she said, "Dr. Koh, the pelvis aligning dance is unbelievable. I could feel its effect right away and it is so fun, dancing to the music. Searching online, I downloaded all your dance instructions shown on TV. Now all my family members are doing it too."

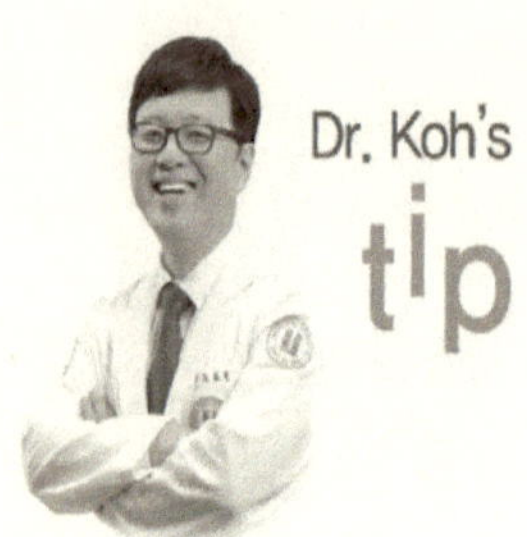



**Pelvic deviation self-diagnosis check list**

. You feel more comfortable while lying on one side compared to the other.

. You feel more comfortable crossing your legs to only one side.

. You have a habitual sprain in one ankle only.

. While sitting on your knees, you often sit and tilt to one side.

. When you buy pants and fit equal lengths, only one side of your pants is always longer.

. You feel comfortable while sitting askew.

. You have different shoulder heights.

. You have a leg length difference.

. From the back, you have a hip height difference.

. There is a big difference between the heels on the right and left side of your shoes that have worn down.

. When you put your feet together and stand upright, there is a space between the inner thighs.

## 02

# LEG LENGTH DISCREPANCY CORRECTING DANCE

 Synopsis

Leg length discrepancy (where one leg is longer than the other) doesn't cause pain if it is less than 2cm, but may result in injury or other problems. There are two types of discrepancies. One is an anatomical discrepancy that is a congenital deformity and another is a physiological discrepancy in which the legs appear to have different lengths due to pelvic deviation when the legs themselves are actually the same length.

Leg Length Discrepancy Correcting Dance is prescribed to improve the physiological discrepancy. In fact, leg length differences are very common some signs of a discrepancy are that the heels of your shoes or the cuffs of your trousers are excessively worn down on one side.

It is important to be aware of the discrepancy and align your body in advance because the discrepancy may have a greater adverse effect on your body than just the problem of the heels of your shoes or the cuffs of your trousers. If you continue to ignore the discrepancy, your body may become misaligned, which may result in the acceleration of a herniated disc or degenerative joint disease, eventually requiring surgery.

The discrepancy causes spinal disorders or joint problems because the pelvic bone tilts superiorly or inferiorly, not laterally. The pelvic tilt results from the movement of the bone above the sacroiliac joint. If you sit cross legged or have incorrect posture, you will get the discrepancy due to the tilted pelvic bone.

When the back of the pelvis drops, the front of the pelvis rises and the femur also rises. Then you have a short leg. In contrast, when the back of the pelvis rises, the front of the pelvis drops. Then you have a long leg.

Therefore, in order to correct your discrepancy, you have to put the back of the pelvis up when the front of the pelvis rises and you have to put the back of the pelvis down when the opposite happens. The Leg Length Discrepancy Correcting Dance is the movements using this principle.

There are some people that want to make both legs long through alignment in order to look taller. This is not recommended. If you try to adjust short legs to long legs even though your pelvis is normal, the alignment can cause abnormalities in your body and lead to more serious problems.

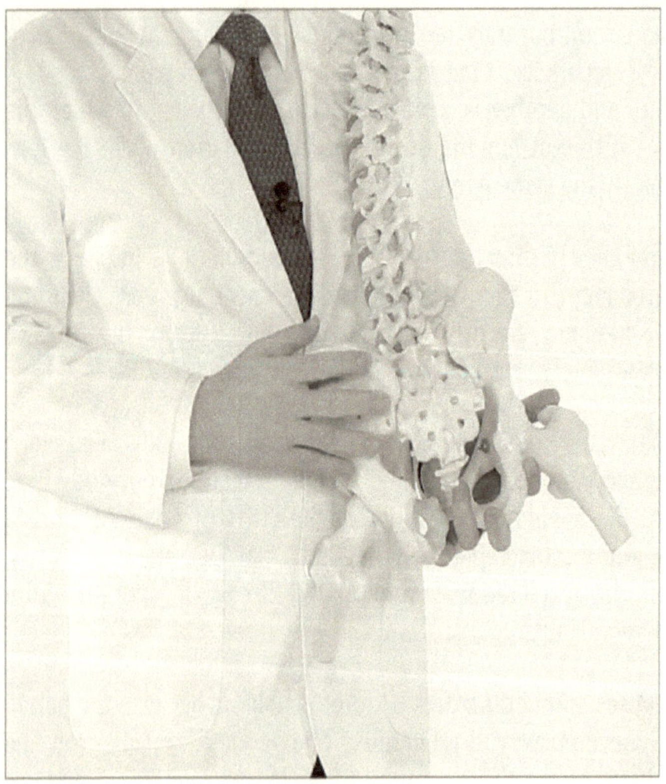

Before the Leg Length Discrepancy Correcting Dance, a required step is the diagnosis of a leg length discrepancy. It is impossible to make the diagnosis by yourself and you will need help from another person.

First, spread a mat on the floor and lie face down. Touch your forehead to the floor and do not rotate your head. Bend your ankles and touch your toes to the floor. Then check both leg lengths at the heels. You will know which leg is shorter or longer.

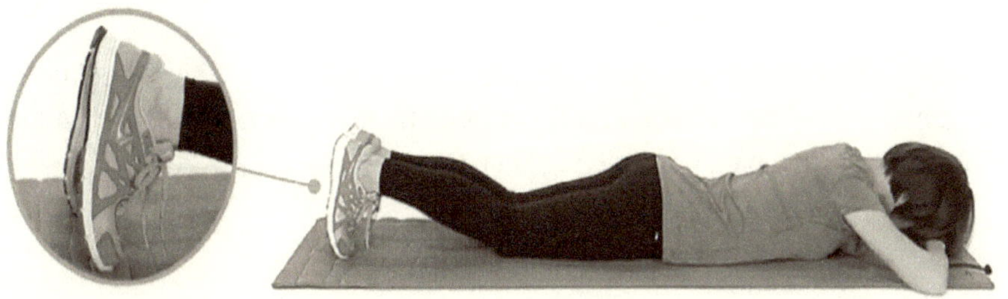

For the case where the right leg is shorter (the left leg is longer)

If your right leg is shorter, you have to put the back of your right pelvis up because the back of your pelvis has dropped. Stand upright and raise your right knee forward. Then straighten the knee backward. This movement will allow you to use the gluteus maximus muscle and help the back of your pelvis rise through the sacroiliac joint. Repeat the above movement 10 times.

If your right leg is shorter, then your left one is longer. So you have to get your longer leg back into place again in order for it to return to normal. The longer leg means that the back of your left pelvis has rised and the front of the pelvis has dropped.

Therefore, you have to put the back of your left pelvis down so that both legs can have the same length. For that reason, you need to raise the left leg towards the chest and lower it. Repeat the movement 10 times. You should maintain the knee angle at about 90 degrees.

After you have aligned both legs, lie face down again and check if both legs have the same length.

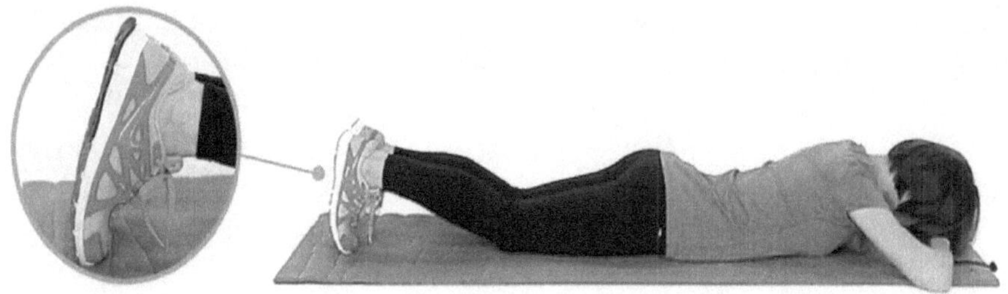

For the case where both legs have the same length

Even if the lengths of both legs became equal, the effect of the correction is sustained only about 3 hours. So it is more effective when you complete the Leg Length Discrepancy Correcting Dance every day.

 Who needs this?

Those who may not have any symptoms but have the discrepancy or the signs mentioned earlier need this dance.

 Basic Movement

Short leg correcting movement

Extend your shorter leg backward, stepping on the ground. Then using the rebounding force, pull the leg forward right away and kick the knee forward. Again, extend the leg backward and step on the ground. You shouldn't kick the knee to the front too much. Slightly bend the other leg and lightly hop at the same spot. Repeat 10 times consecutively.

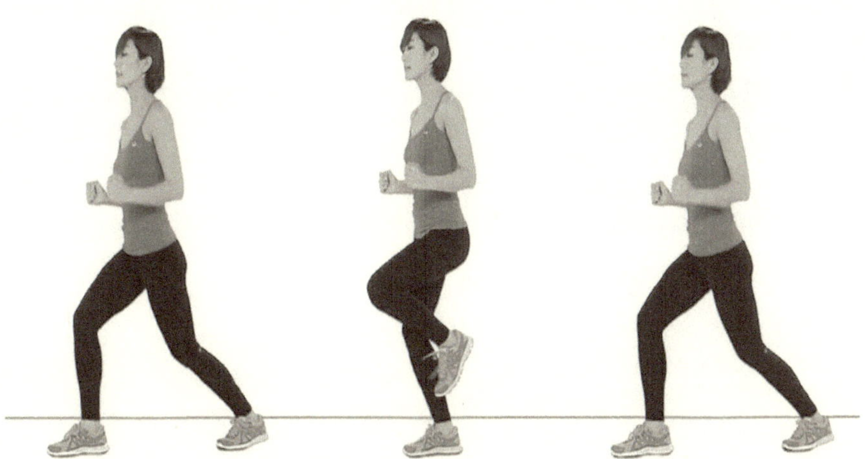

## Long leg correcting movement

Lift up your longer leg, bending the knee to a right angle and then bring it down to the ground. Repeat the movement 10 times.

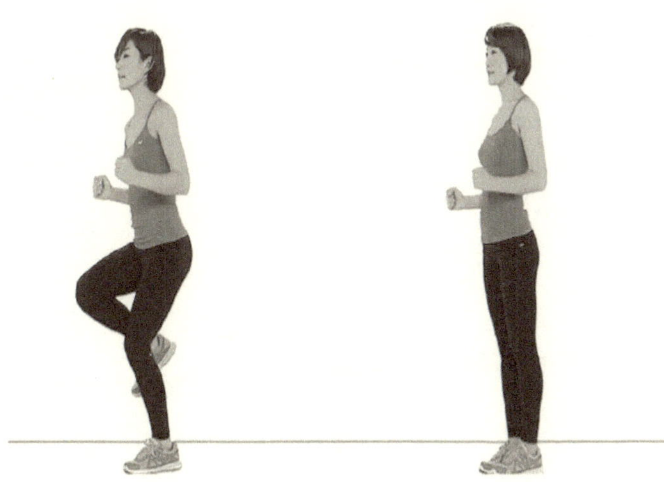

1. After checking the length of your legs, stand at attention. Naturally place both arms to the sides in a right angle.

2. Bend the left knee if your left leg is shorter, the right knee if your right leg is shorter.

3. Straighten the bent knee, pulling the leg backward and dip the toes on the ground. Repeat #2 and #3 10 times.

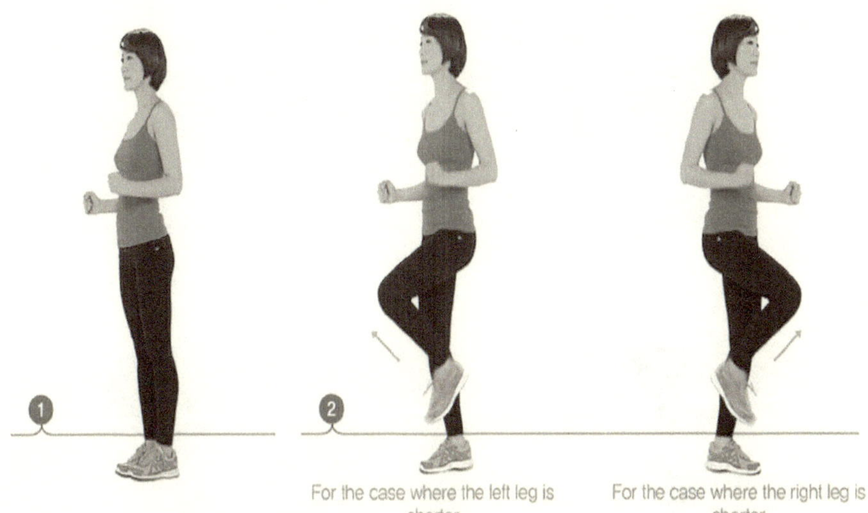



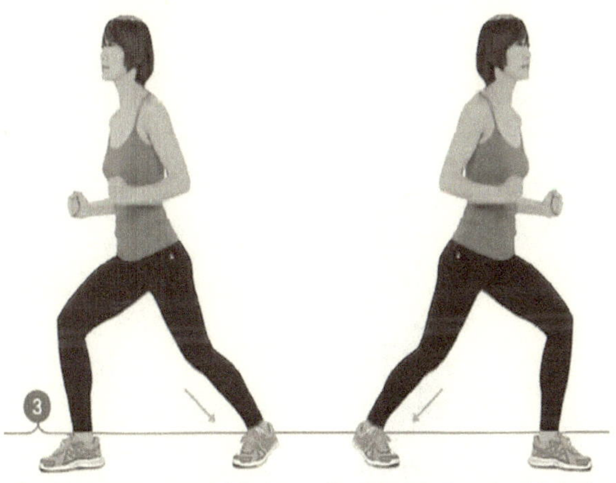



## Long leg correcting movement

4 Lift up the other leg and bend knee to 90 degrees.

5 Stralghten the bent knee to the ground. Repeat #4 and #5 10 times. Then check the leg length difference through self-diagnosis. If the legs are not aligned yet, repeat #2~5 till they are aligned.

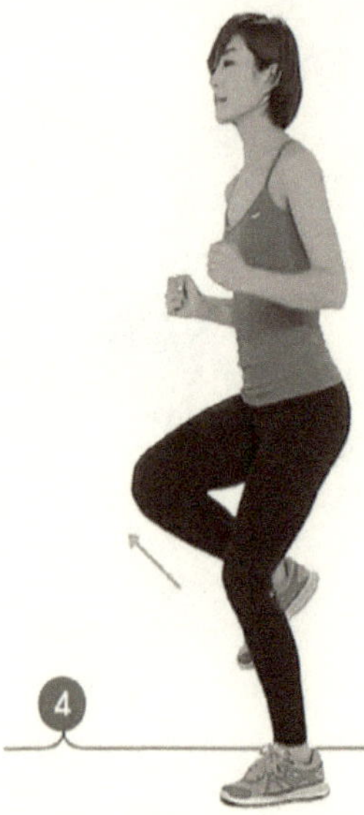 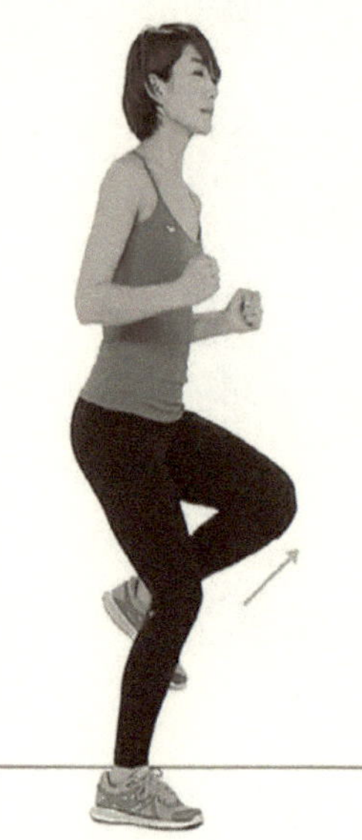

For the case where the right leg is longer | For the case where the left leg is longer

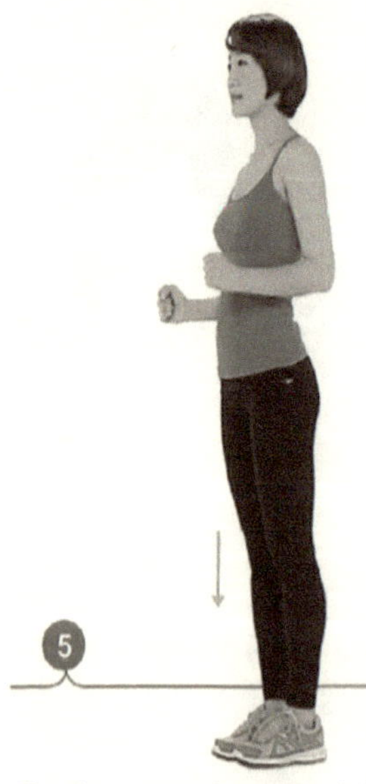 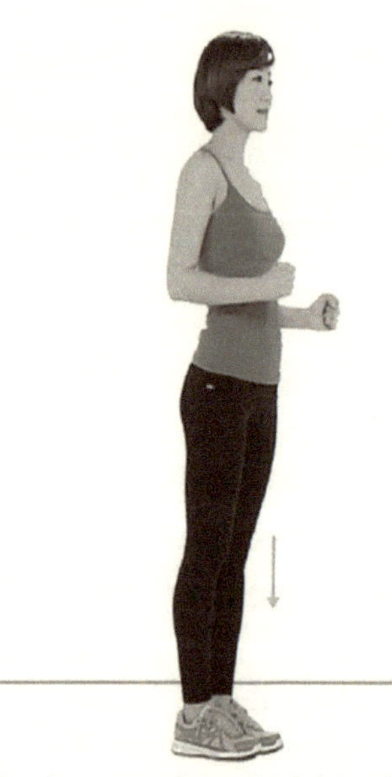

For the case where the right leg is longer | For the case where the left leg is longer

The biggest effect of this dance is the correction of a leg length discrepancy.



The exercise is for correcting the discrepancy, but this isn't a one time cure. You have to check your leg length regularly and do the exercise consistently in order to prevent the discrepancy.



Mr. A is an elderly gentleman in his 60s who has been treated in my hospital for a slipped disc. One day during the course of care, Mr. A asked, "Dr. Koh, would the leg length get different when you have disc disease?" When I asked why he was curious, he replied that he has observed that one side of his pants felt longer than the other side, so he searched online and performed a self-diagnosis and found out that his right leg was shorter.

Mr. A seemed to believe that all those signs were caused by the slipped disc. He was worried that his right leg will continue to get shorter and that he will need to get surgery to extend the leg.

After explaining to Mr. A about the uneven legs, I taught him the Leg Length discrepancy Correcting Dance. Mr. A visited me a few weeks later and said, "Thanks to you, my wife and I got hooked into dancing."

His wife was skeptical at first, telling him what's up with dancing at an old age, but after listening to Mr. A's explanation, she started dancing with him. To help this couple live a healthier life, I taught them the other dance movements.

At the next visit, Mr. A said, "All my family members got into dancing thanks to you!," and laughed. He liked how he and his wife could listen to their favorite songs and do the Spine Health Dance.

He taught the dance to his children who were lacking exercise because of their busy daily lives and now all the family members are dancing together. His children told their friends about the effect of this dance too, so now the Spine Health Dance has become popular among people around Mr. A.

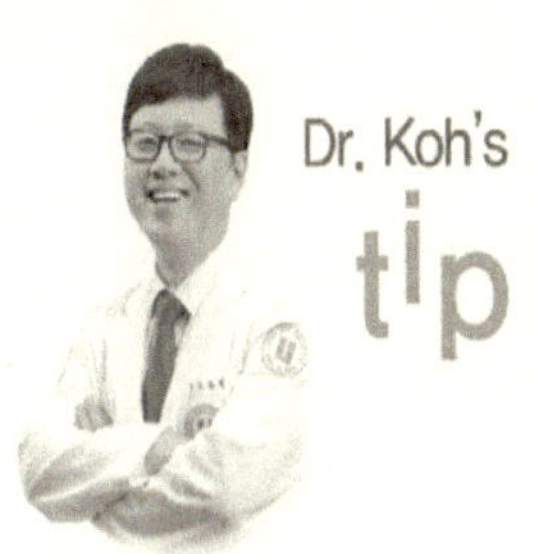


**The correcting method of the complex pelvic problems**
Complex pelvic problems are the leg length discrepancy with a tilted pelvis. For example, when you close your eyes, walk in place for 40 steps, and your body leans toward the right, then your pelvis has been tilted to the right. Also, your right leg is shorter when you lie face down and check your leg length.

In this case, first correct the shorter right leg in order to make both leg lengths same. Then close your eyes, walk in place for 40 steps again, and check if your pelvis is aligned. If you make both leg lengths same, your tilted pelvis should usually move back into place.

If your pelvis has been aligned, you don't need any other correction. However, if your pelvis is still tilted to the right, you can align the right side of your pelvic through the Pelvic Alignment Dance. For the opposite case where your left leg is shorter and the left side of your pelvis is tilted, the correction method is same.

If your left leg is shorter and the right side of your pelvis is tilted, first correct the shorter left leg and then align the tilted right pelvis. In other words, after you correct the shorter leg, do self diagnosis, and if your problem has not been fixed, then complete the Pelvic Alignment Dance.

When you correct the shorter leg, do not forget to correct not only the shorter leg but the other longer leg as well.

# FORWARD
# NECK
## DANCE

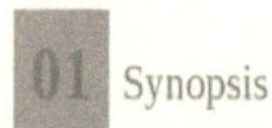 Synopsis

Ordinarily, the cervical spine has a forward curve (c shaped), the thoracic spine has a backward curve (reverse c shaped), and the lumbar spine has a forward curve (c shaped). A forward neck is anteriorly translocated from its normal c position, and it causes pain around the neck, headaches, and shoulder pain. The biggest cause of the forward neck syndrome is poor posture. If the anterior positioning of the cervical spine is maintained continuously, the upper spine will get stressed and the muscles and ligaments on the back of the neck will be pulled, which causes pain.

Actually, almost every posture in our routine lives is putting the arms forward and flexing the neck. When sitting down and studying at a desk, working at the office, driving a car, and washing the dishes, people are prone to a forward posture. Nowadays, people also use smartphones in the same posture even while walking on the street.

Even when the head is translocated forward one centimeter, the cervical spine receives an additional load of 4~7 pounds weight. At first, the weight is inappreciable, but over time you may have difficulty concentrating experience whole body fatigue, shoulder discomfort, neck pain, headaches, vertigo, numbness in hands, and/or eye strain.

The Forward Neck Dance is the opposite of the usual poor posture. You have to send your arms backward and extend your neck in order to make its normal c curve. However, it doesn't work if you only extend your neck.

Looking at the upper body from the side, the neck and the low back curve slightly inward and the mid back curves outward. These three natural curves give the upper body an S shape. It becomes a problem when it is twisted out of shape and into a forward neck. Therefore, when you open the chest using your arms, you maintain the backward curve of the thoracic spine in order to return the neck to its normal position.

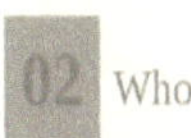

## 02  Who needs this?

Those who experience symptoms such as difficulty concentrating, whole body fatigue, shoulder discomfort, neck pain, headaches, vertigo, numbness in the hands, eye strain, and so on and those who are diagnosed with forward neck syndrome will benefit from the dance.

## 03  Basic Movement

The basic movement of the Forward Neck Dance originates from the basic movement of the Electronic Dance, but the difference is in sending the arms backward to widely open the chest. At the start of the dance, lift the arms to the height of the chest and bend them in an L shape. Then send the arms backward using shoulders as you pull out the buttocks backward as you, bend the knees. Send the arms completely backward to the point where the chest is fully opened and the back muscles get tight.

Straighten the knees and bring back the arms to the original position. As you repeat this movement, gradually increase the pace when you get into the rhythm. This is a continuous movement, using the rebounding force from the pelvis.

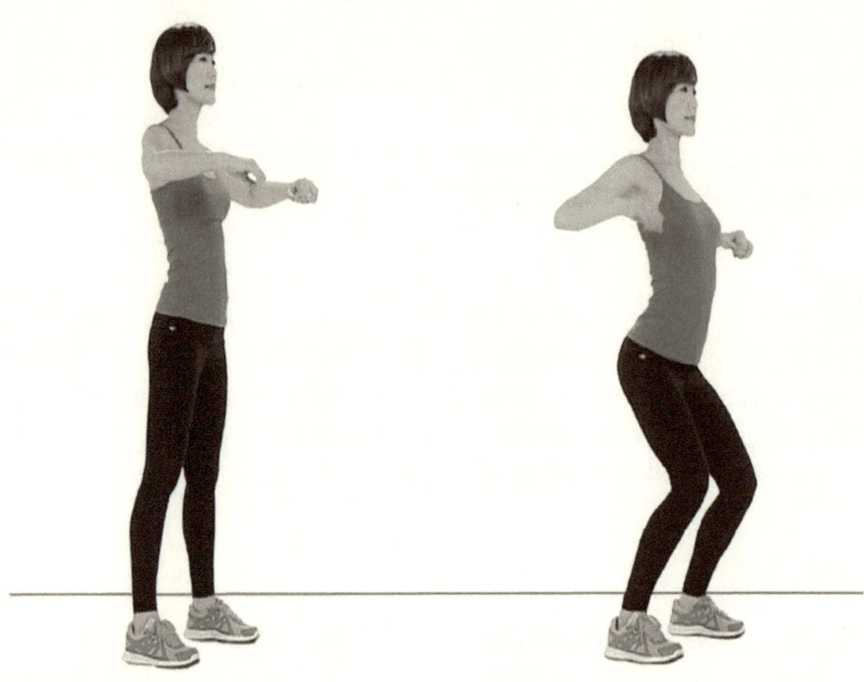



1 Stand with the legs shoulder width apart. Lift the arms and bend the elbows in an L shape.

2 Bend the knees while tightening the core and making the waist C shaped. As you pull out the buttocks backward, strongly pull the arms backward to open the chest.

3 Bring the arms back to the original position as you stand up. Repeat #2~3.

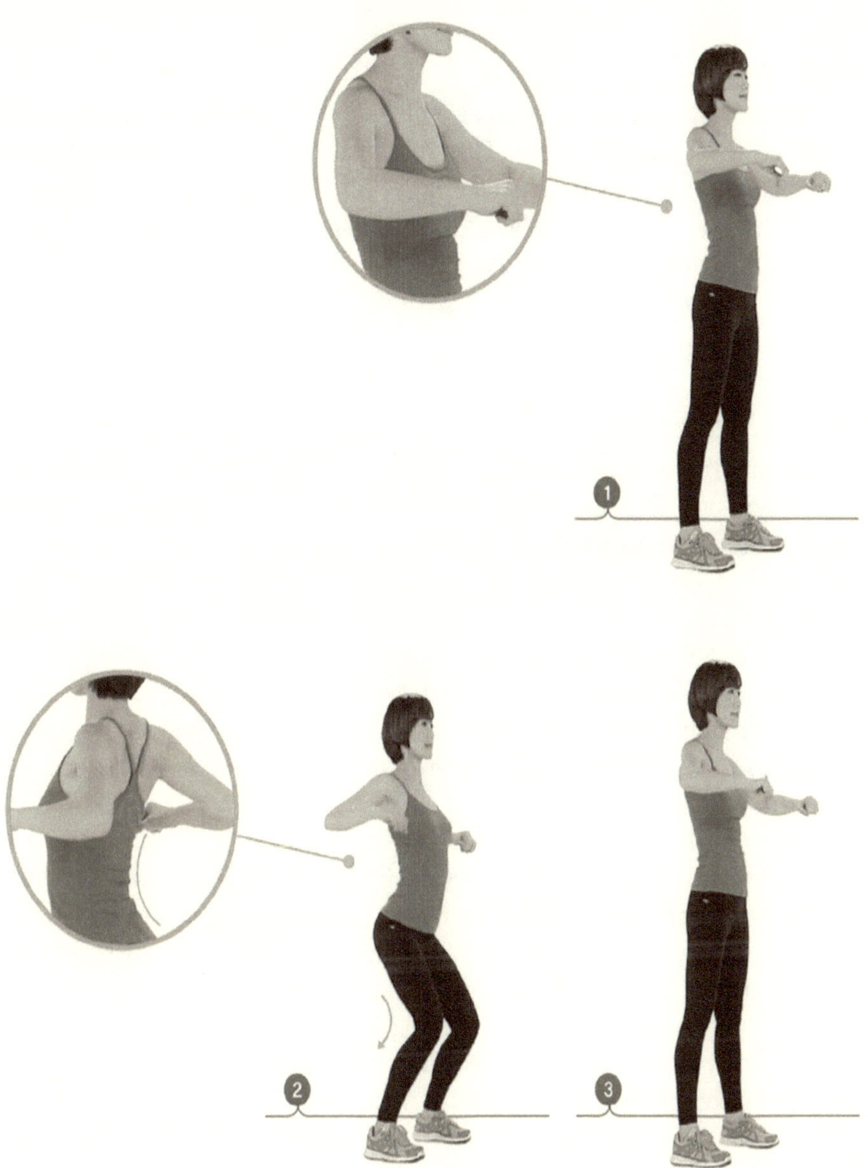





The biggest effect is the improvement of the forward neck posture and the exercise can also prevent the recurrence of the forward neck syndrome by poor posture which can't be improved easily in daily life.

**06** Caution

The movements of the dance look simple, but they have an influence on the neck, the waist, and the knees. Therefore, make sure to spend enough time warming-up, such as stretching the neck, massaging the back of the neck fully, stretching (rotating) the waist, and bending and straightening the knees before the dance. This makes the exercise safe and maximizes its effects. (Refer to "Stretching")

**07** Example

Mr. O, an office worker in his 40s, came to me suffering from chronic fatigue and muscle pain throughout the whole body. Mr. O's spine seemed to be in danger because of his work environment of sitting along with a high pressure job.

The pain in his neck and shoulders constantly tormented Mr. O, especially near the end of his work day. He told me that he also found it difficult to drive back home because of migraines and eye fatigue. After getting home, he felt so tired that he couldn't even have a conversation with his family members.

Due to his symptoms. I talked about the Spine Health Dance and gave him the dance instructions on a CD, and said, "Give it a try. When your body becomes healthy, you will be able to overcome fatigue and at least alleviate the pain in your spine caused by your work environment."

Having received the CD, Mr. O seemed somewhat doubtful. I understood that he might have felt that what I told him was a little absurd. Telling someone who was too exhausted to even have a conversation with his family to dance. I hoped that he would try the Spine Health Dance little by little.

Mr. O who visited me at least once every few weeks to a month came to me 2 months later. He seemed more energetic than before and did not seem exhausted. When I asked if there were any good news, he replied, "It's because you have given me the best medicine. At first I thought, 'Why did Dr. Koh tell me to do such a difficult thing?,' but I came to like it and although I can't get into the rhythm that well, being a bad dancer, I danced every day as I got somewhat addicted to dancing with music."

It was clearly noticeable, Mr. O's forward neck syndrome was significantly improved. All the pain that had pressed him down was gone as his spine and neck were better aligned. I feel indescribably rewarded whenever I receive positive feedback on my Spine Health Dance.

# 4



# Joint Strengthening Dance

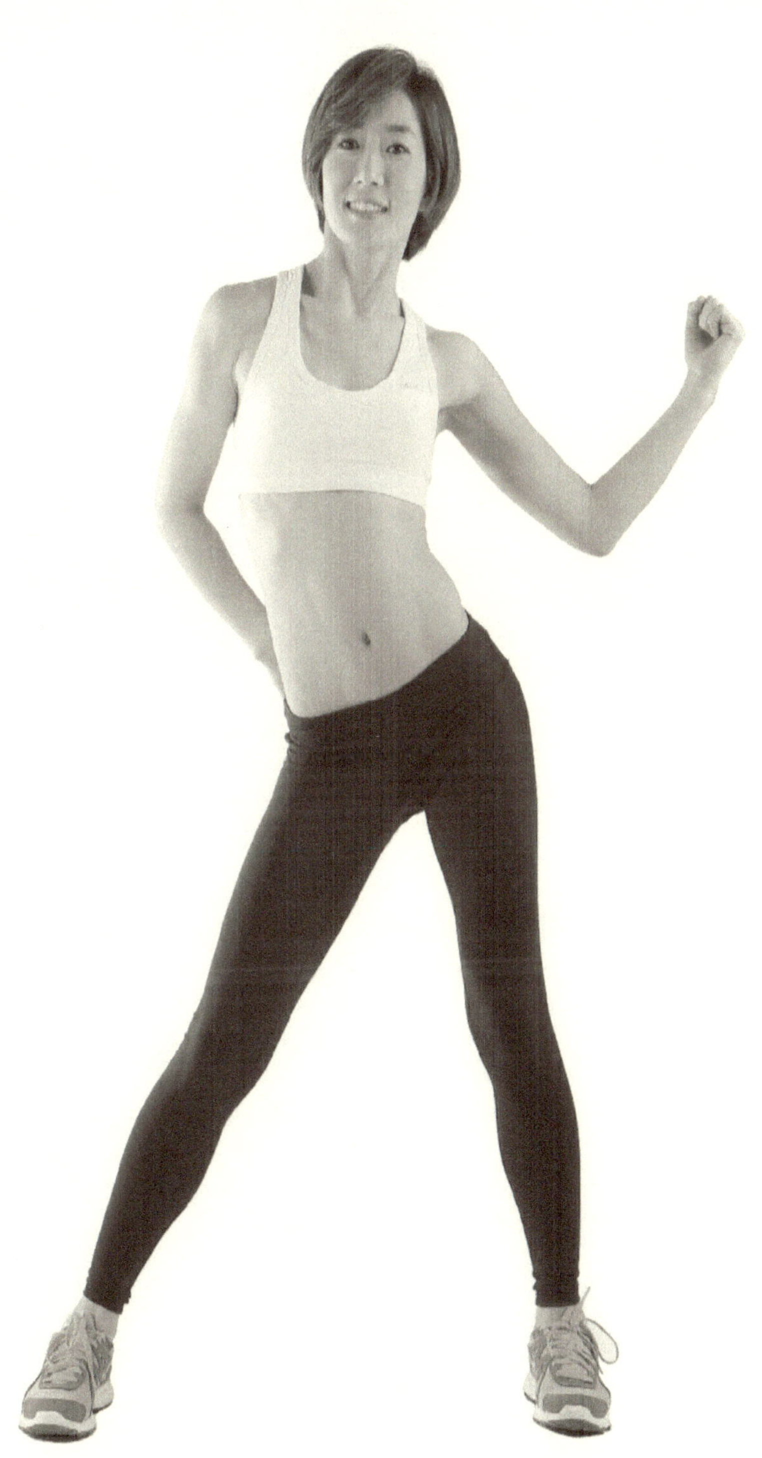

I would like to introduce the dance for protecting joints. Using side core, shoulder and arm muscles that you don't use often, you can safely strengthen the muscles and stabilize the muscles around joints when you perform these dances consistently.

# 01
# WHIRLWIND
## DANCE

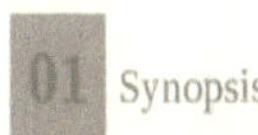 Synopsis

The Whirlwind Dance allows patients to strengthen the shoulder muscles and the side core muscles that they don't use often which can get injured easily. If these muscles are strengthened, it can help prevent upper body and shoulder problems.

**02** Who needs this?

This exercise can help someone who has shoulder pain or a weak upper body. The dance allows patients to strengthen their shoulder and upper body muscles and is also good for those who need a full body workout.

**03 Basic Movement**

Stand with legs shoulder width apart, raise the right arm forward as if you are bowling, and slightly lift the left leg and put it on the ground as you push the pelvis to the left. At this point, put your weight on the left leg.
Then, move your weight to the other side. raise the left arm forward, slightly lift the right leg and put it on the ground as you push the pelvis to the right. Repeat this movement.

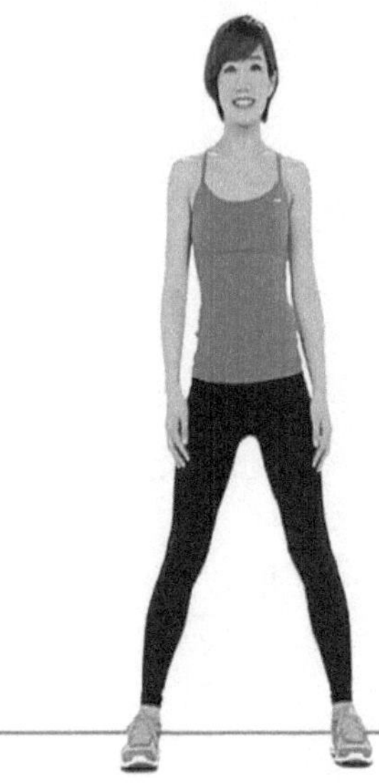



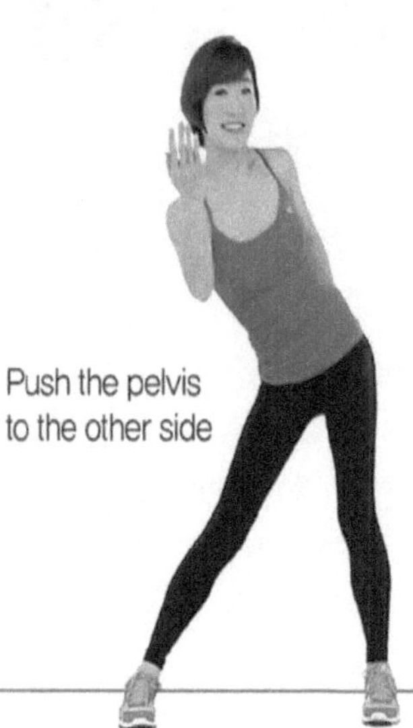



## 04 Details

1 Stand with legs shoulder width apart.

2 Raise the right arm forward as if you are bowling and slightly lift the left leg simultaneously.

3 As you put the left leg on the ground, push the pelvis to the left at the same time. Put your weight on the left leg.

4 Raise the left arm forward as in #2 and slightly lift the right leg simultaneously.

5 Just like in #3, as you put the right leg on the ground, push the pelvis to the right at the same time. Put your weight on the right leg. Repeat #2~5.

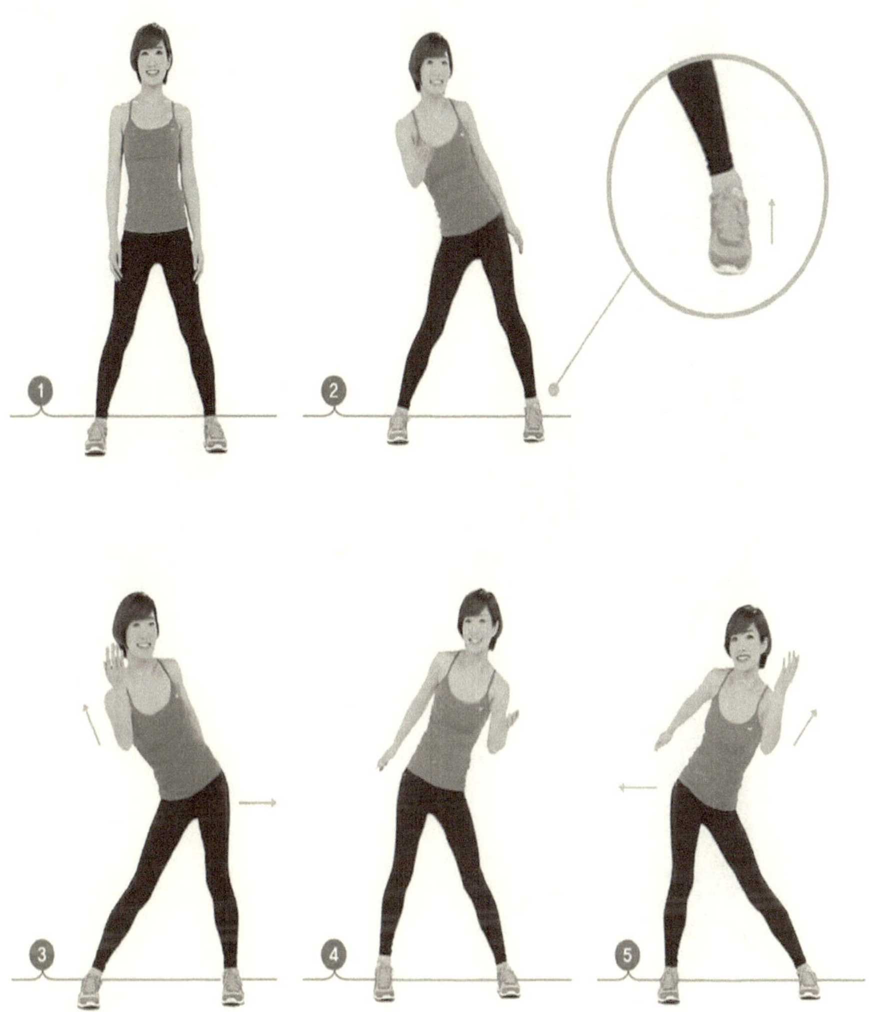



Basically any dance is a full body workout. The Whirlwind Dance activates the oblique abdominal muscle, the quadratus lumborum muscle, and the latissimus dorsi muscle in the trunk when you raise the arm forward as if you are bowling, and also stimulates the biceps brachii muscle and the triceps brachii muscle when you stretch the arm.

When you pull out the buttocks from side to side, the gluteus medius muscle, the gluteus maximus muscle, and the sacroiliac joints are strengthened. When you hold the legs tight, thigh muscles such as the quadriceps femoris muscle are strengthened.

When you raise the arm forward, you have the effect of pulling the same side flank muscles and stretching the other side. If your side muscles are strengthened, you will slim down naturally and most of all, they will help support the spine strongly. Then you will have a healthy body.

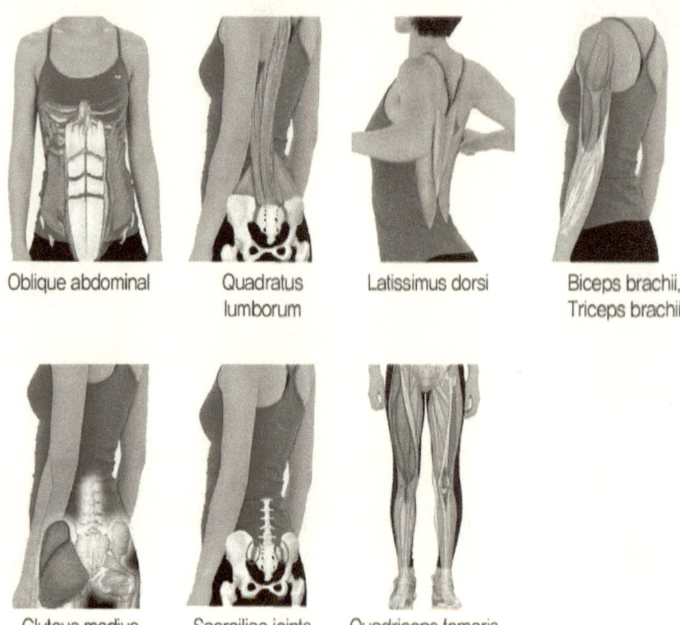

Oblique abdominal

Quadratus lumborum

Latissimus dorsi

Biceps brachii, Triceps brachii

Gluteus medius, Gluteus maximus

Sacroiliac joints

Quadriceps femoris

06 Caution

Because the Whirlwind Dance is the exercise for muscles that you don't use often, make sure to spend enough time to warm-up in order to stretch the side and shoulder muscles before the dance. (Refer to "Stretching")

07 Example

Mr. M, a baseball enthusiast and a batter on his team, is an office worker in his 40s. He was a patient who was passionate about playing baseball to the extent where he had a history of an oblique strain requiring 3 weeks of rehabilitation.

When Mr. M visited me again from his far away hometown for his mother and mother-in-law's disc condition, I gave him the Spine Health Dance CD after finding out that he got injured with an oblique strain last year. Mr. M smiled bashfully and with a doubtful face saying, "Did you say that a dance can help with realigning and rehabilitation?"

After a few months, Mr. M came back with his mother. I wanted to ask if he is following the Spine Health Dance, but couldn't as I remembered his facial expression when he received the CD. I thought Mr. M wouldn't do it just because of the fact that it is a dance.

When his mother's course of care was completed, Mr. M smiled and said, "Dr. Koh, my baseball team is doing your Spine Health Dance as a warm-up exercise these days. I was a little shy to do it in front of my wife or kids, so I suggested to my baseball team members to do it together and they started dancing with me out of curiosity. I thought it was nothing, but it really was a good exercise. Some team members started doing it with their family too. The kids were enthusiastic about dancing. I'm focusing on the dance for my sides because I realized the importance of side muscles and because it feel good on my sides after doing it. I wanted to say thank you."

One of my acquaintances who reads and writes books all the time suffered from not only back and shoulder pain but also pain in the sides. Because he was a guy who never exercises, I taught him the Whirlwind Dance and suggested that he consider it to be a part of listening to music and try the dance whenever reading or writing gets boring.

Taking a look at the first movement, he laughed and said, "Why don't you just tell me to go bowling instead?" When I insisted, telling him to trust me on this one, he mumbled, "You are telling me to dance when exercising is the last thing I would do?"

He must have done the dance pretty hard. Feeling the effect of the dance himself, he then learned the dance movements one by one and now he is even better than me. The Whirlwind Dance became his favorite.

He told me that at first, his entire body particularly his sides hurt, but gradually as time passed, he felt so refreshed and light after the dance that he is dancing whenever he could. He doesn't visit me complaining about the pain in his back or sides anymore.

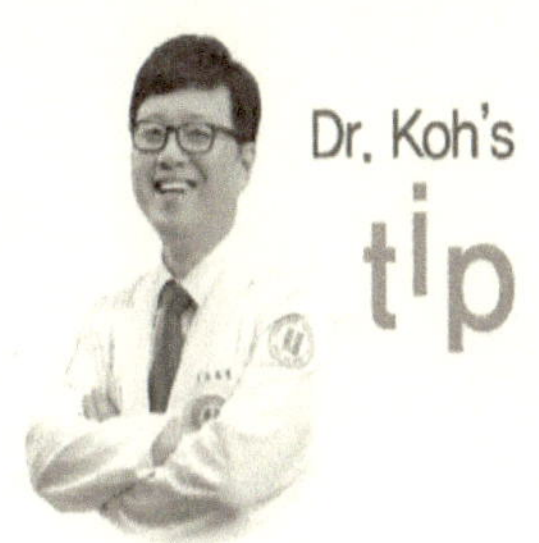



**Triceps brachii muscle**
The triceps brachii muscle is an extensor muscle of the elbow joint on the back of the upper arm and a spindle shaped muscle that runs along the humerus between the shoulder and the forearm. The triceps brachii muscle has three heads, a long head, a lateral head, and a medial head. The long head arises from the lower part of the glenoid cavity on the scapula. The other two heads arise from the upper and lower parts of the groove for radial nerve on the back of the humerus.

**Biceps brachii muscle**
The biceps brachii muscle on the front of the upper arm flexes the forearm at the elbow, supinates the forearm, and is controlled by the musculo- cutaneous nerve. This muscle is known as the biceps due to being a two headed muscle, long head and short head. The short head of the biceps brachii muscle prevents a dislocation of the shoulder joint.

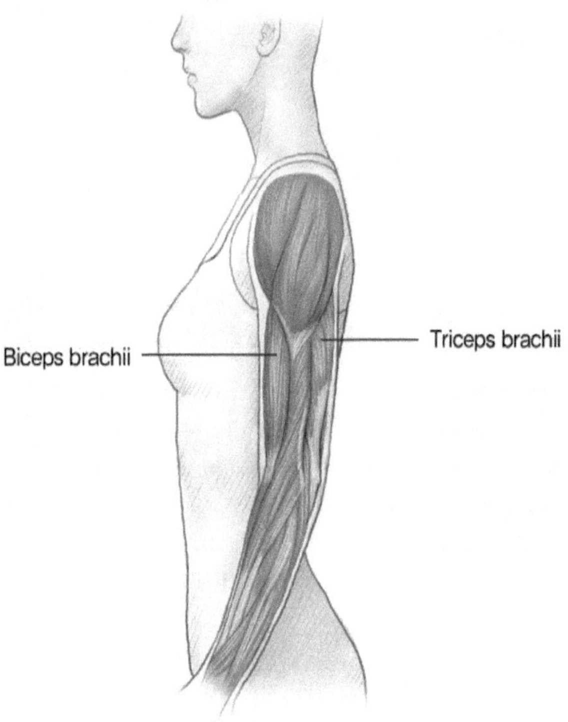

Biceps brachii
Triceps brachii

# 02
# SHOULDER
## DANCE

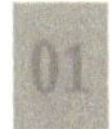 Synopsis

Our shoulders are used constantly but get little exercise. That is why people often suffer from shoulder pain. The Shoulder Dance helps to strengthen the shoulder muscles, prevents pain and frozen shoulder (adhesive capsulitis).

Frozen shoulder, also known as "fifties' shoulder" disease in Korea, gets its korean name from symptoms of the shoulder common in people in their fifties. Now, patients who have adhesive capsulitis of the shoulder tend to be younger because people have various sports activities or use smartphones and computers for long periods of time.

If patients have frozen shoulder, they have intense pain in the shoulder and movements of the shoulder become severely restricted. If you leave it as it is, the pain will be gone but the shoulder will be stiff. In severe cases, patients aren't able to move their fingers and have extreme pain.

 Who needs this?

This dance is to prevent frozen shoulder and also makes patients who have frozen shoulder get better. Those who have other shoulder symptoms such as pain can make their shoulders stronger through this dance.

**03 Basic Movement**

Spread the arms and legs in the shape of a Chinese character '大.' Raise the arms horizontally, making a right angle at the armpit and spread the legs wide. While moving the lower body slightly left and right, push the shoulders left and right in the direction opposite to the lower body movement, considering the pelvis to be the central axis.

When pushing the shoulders to the right, twist the right palm facing up and the left palm facing down. In the opposite movement of the shoulders, change the direction the palms face in.

After the consecutive movements, while raising both arms to the sides and making a right angle at the armpit, bend the elbows to a right angle and lower and raise both hands. Then alternately move the right and left hand up and down.

Repeat these three movements.

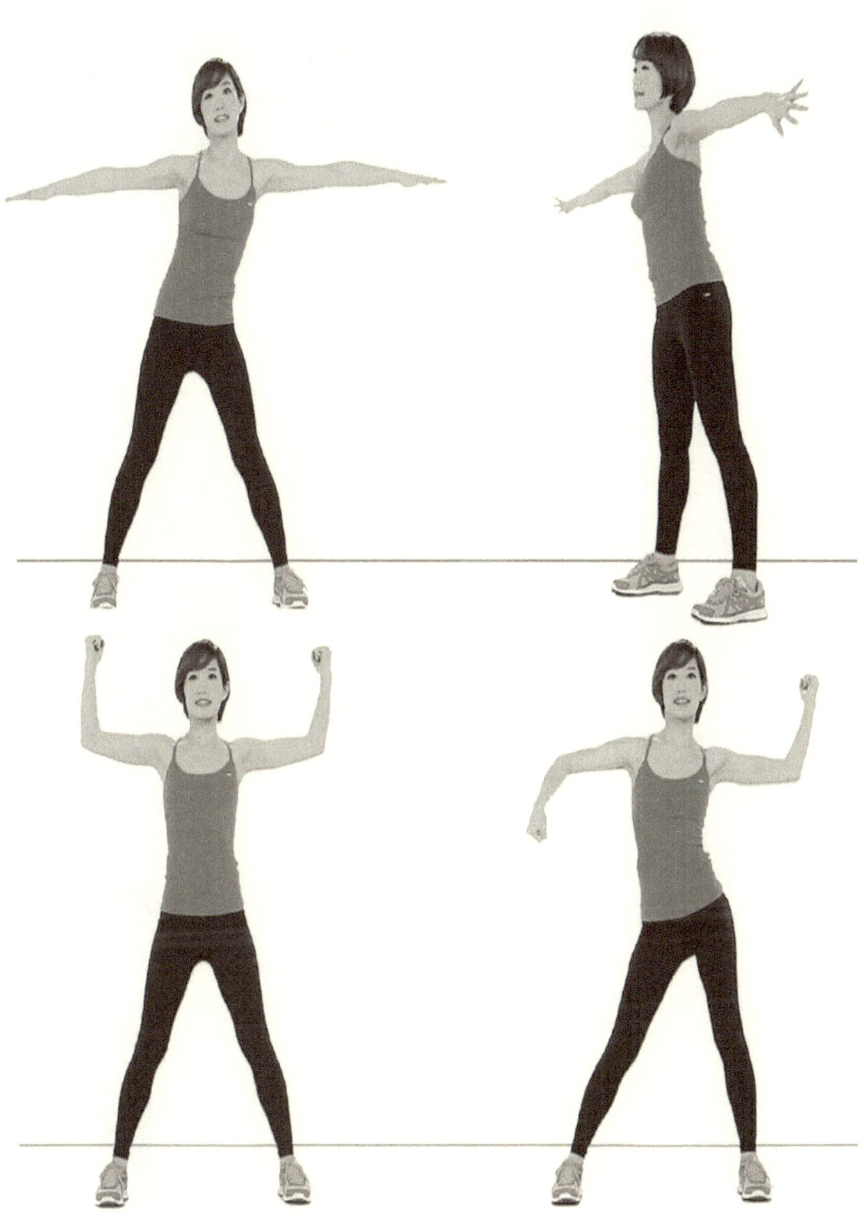



1 Spread both arms horizontally, making a right angle at the armpit and also

spread the legs wide.

2 While moving the lower body slightly left and right, strongly push the shoulders in the direction opposite to the lower body movement.

3 When pushing the shoulders to the right, twist the right palm facing up and the left palm facing down. In the opposite movement, when pushing the shoulders to the left, twist the left palm facing up and the right palm facing down.

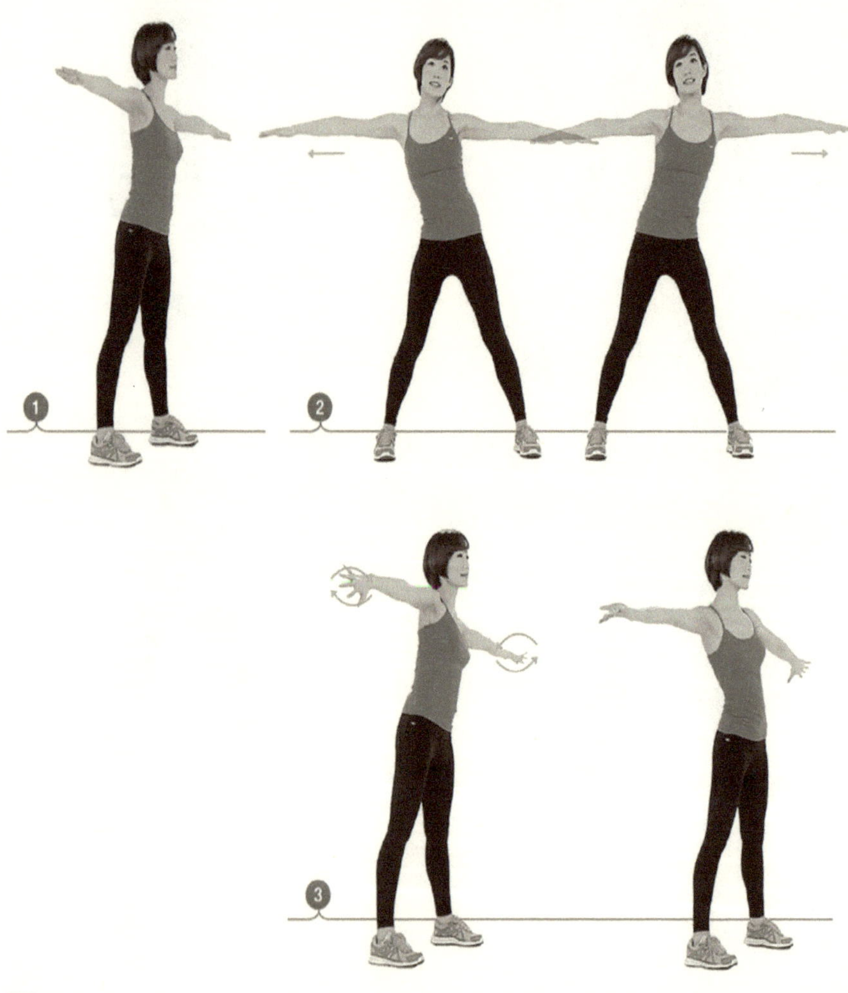

4 With arms raised up horizontally, making a right angle at the armpit, bend

at the elbows to a right angle and lower the hands. Repeat moving both hands up and down.

5 Then, alternately repeat moving the left and right hand up and down. Repeat #2~5 as consecutively.

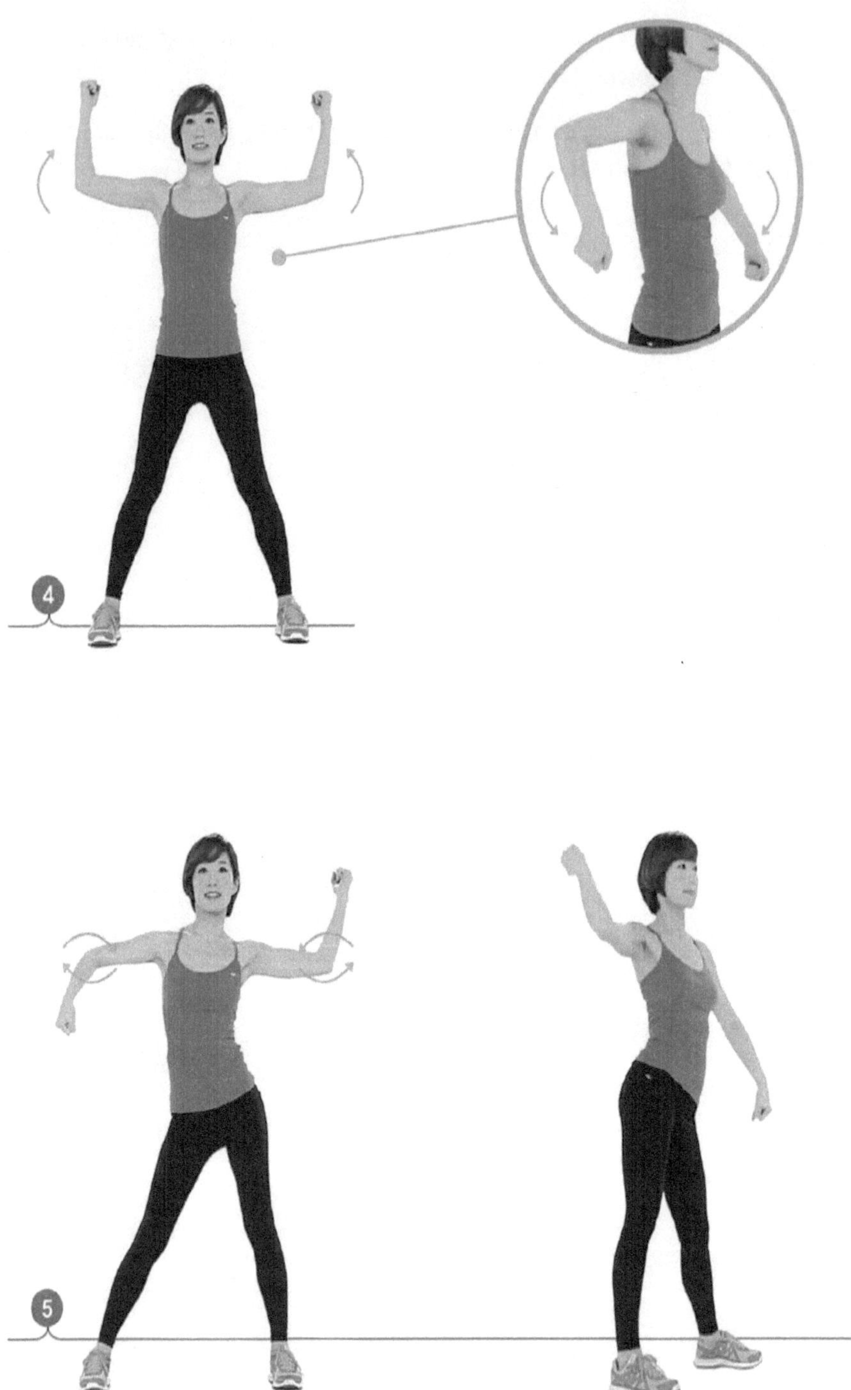

05 Effects

## 05 Effects

When the arms are raised to 45 degrees at the armpit, the supraspinatus muscle is activated and at 90 degrees, the deltoid muscle is activated. In the Shoulder Dance, the deltoid muscle is strengthened because you raise the arms horizontally and twist the arms as much as possible in the direction opposite to each other.

Also, with the arms raised horizontally and bent to 90 degrees, alternately moving the left and right hand up and down will help strengthen the infraspinatus and the subscapularis muscles (Part of your rotator cuff muscles).

## 06 Caution

Because the exercise strains the shoulder and upper body muscles more than it seems, make sure to spend enough time to warm-up before the dance. (Refer to "Stretching") For people with serious frozen shoulder, it is desirable that they get medical advice before completing this dance. People with serious shoulder pain will improve shoulder mobility when they do the dance after receiving a simple treatment in the hospital to relieve the pain.

## 07 Example

One of the hospital employees who had initial symptoms of frozen shoulder started the Shoulder Dance as a skeptic. At first, he felt tremendous pain in his stiff shoulders, but he worked through the pain patiently and continued the dance in order to avoid the shoulders from getting worse.

About a month later, the pain and difficulties from movements were gone and the shoulders that felt so heavy gradually became lighter. This employee is now learning other Spine Health Dance movements.

After experiencing relief from shoulder pain, he now plans to learn the other movements to get healthier. He prefers the Spine Health Dance to other exercises because he could do it without getting restricted on time or location.

To the five patients who came to my clinic suffering from frozen shoulder pain, I taught them the Shoulder Dance and had them consistently perform the dance. The results were amazing. After treating the pain with an injection, patients told me that their pain gradually reduced and/or their range of motion got better within a couple weeks.

I had twelve patients suffering from other types of shoulder pain than frozen shoulder. When I had them do the Shoulder Dance, 100% of them had their shoulder pain gone in a short time varying from a few days to a few weeks and maintained the painless condition. moreover, as the result of the dance, the patients felt light and did not feel overloaded on their arms or shoulders even after long work hours on a computer.

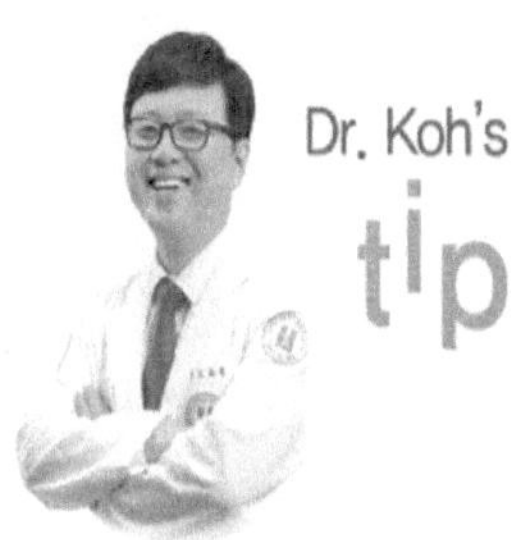



**Trapezius muscle**

The trapezius muscle extends longitudinally from the occipital bone to the lower thoracic spine and laterally to the scapula and its functions are to move the shoulder and support the arm.

The muscle is divided into three regions. The upper region elevates the scapula, the middle region retracts the scapula, and the lower region depresses the scapula.

**Deltoid muscle**

The deltoid muscle has an important role to stabilize the glenohumeral joint (shoulder joint) and consists of three muscles (anterior deltoid, lateral [middle] deltoid, and posterior deltoid). The muscle needs to be strong in order to prevent a dislocation of the shoulder. This muscle abducts the shoulder.

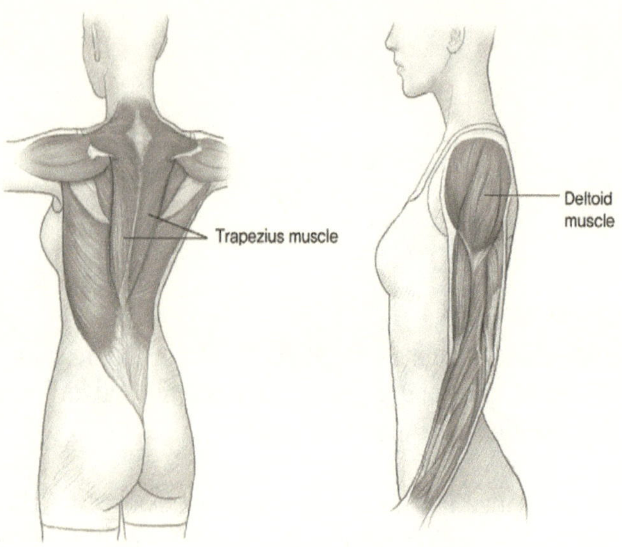



## Subscapularis muscle

The subscapularis muscle is located on the underside of the scapula, passes the front of the humeral head, and inserts into the lesser tubercle of the humerus. The function of the muscle is to stabilize the humeral head of the glenohumeral joint and internally rotate the humerus.

## Infraspinatus muscle

The infraspinatus muscle is part of the rotator cuff which also includes the supraspinatus muscle, the teres minor muscle, and the subscapularis muscle. The muscle externally rotates the humerus and stabilizes the shoulder joint during the arm movement.

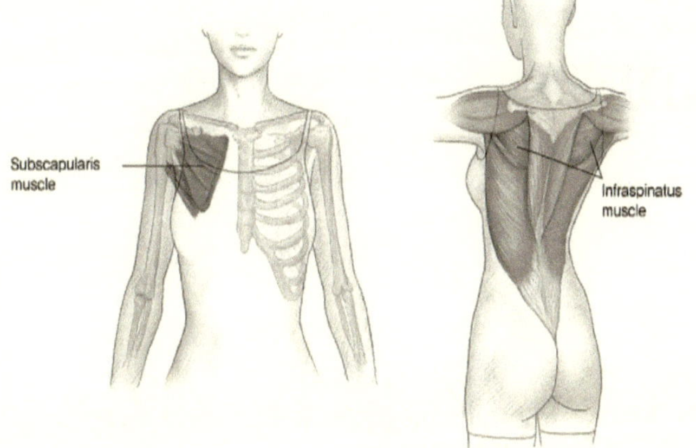


Subscapularis
muscle
Infraspinatus
muscle

# 03
# **HANDLE**
# DANCE

 Synopsis

The handle Dance is also for strengthening the shoulders, so the effect of the dance is similar to that of the Shoulder Dance. This one is less strain on the shoulders than the Shoulder Dance so that people with weaker shoulders can easily perform this dance. Also, the movements are interesting as they are simple and fun.

Just like its name, the Handle Dance involves a movement that mimics steering a wheel and a hand twisting movement like the dance move in a K-Pop song 'Choryun' by Clon. These movements are easy and fun, making the dance enjoyable while strengthening the shoulders.

 Who needs this?

This dance is for anybody who feel like their shoulders are weak. As it prevents pain in the shoulders by strengthening them, it is certainly a necessary therapy for the people who use their shoulders a lot at work or the people who spend a long time in front of a computer.

**03 Basic Movement**

Sway the pelvis left and right to the rhythm, lifting the arm on the side of the pelvic movement direction and lowering the other arm behind the buttocks. As you swing the pelvis, use the rebounding force from alternating both arms to twist the shoulders.
While swaying the pelvis, raise both arms forward and clench the fists as if you are holding onto a wheel. Twist the entire arms from the shoulders to the

hands as if you are twisting the wheel in the direction of the pelvic movement. The point here is to fully straighten the arms forward.
With both arms fully extended, cross over the wrists, open the fists, and twist them left and right in the direction of the pelvic movement.

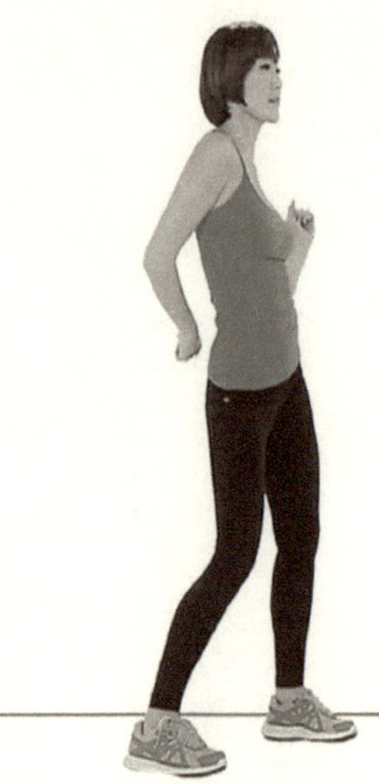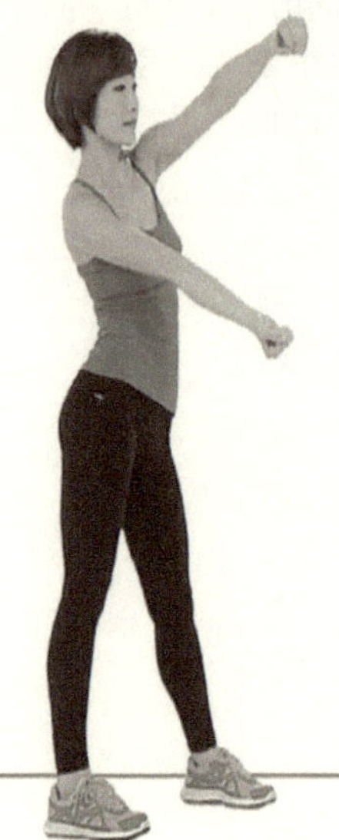

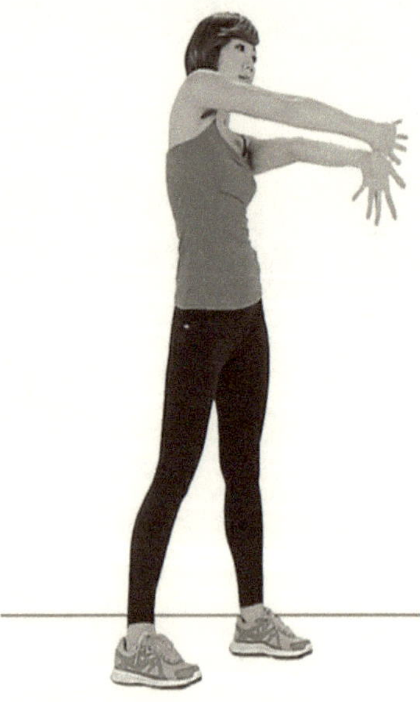

1 Swaying the pelvis left and right, lift the arm on the side of the direction of the pelvic movement and lower the other arm behind the buttocks.

2 While swaying the pelvis, raise both arms forward, clench the fists as if you are holding onto a wheel and twist the arms like driving in the direction of the pelvic movement.

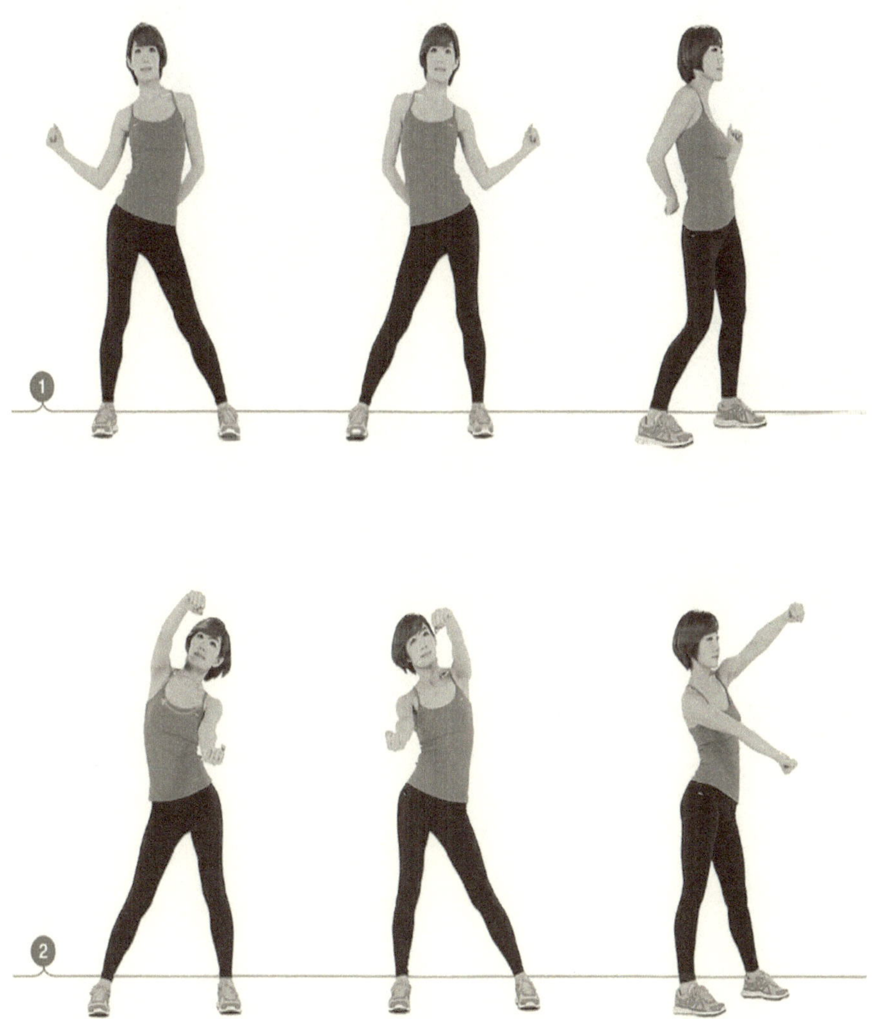

3 While swaying the pelvis, cross over the wrists, open the fists, and twist

them left and right in the direction of the pelvic movement. Repeat #1~3.

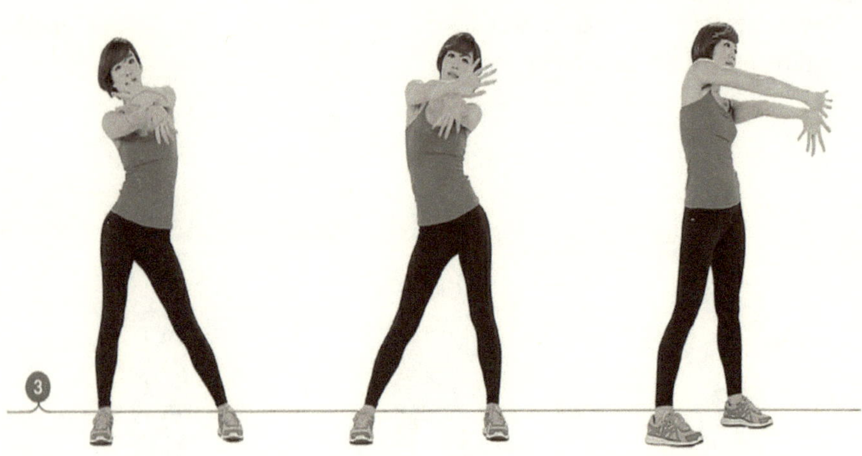

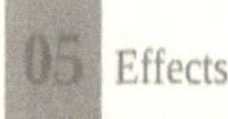


The Handle Dance makes the shoulder muscles, especially the infraspinatus and the subscapularis muscles, stronger.

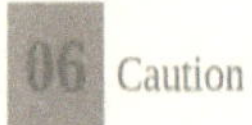


Because there is a lot of movement of the shoulder muscles in this dance, make sure to spend enough time to warm-up before the dance in order to prepare the shoulder muscles. (Refer to "Stretching")

# 5

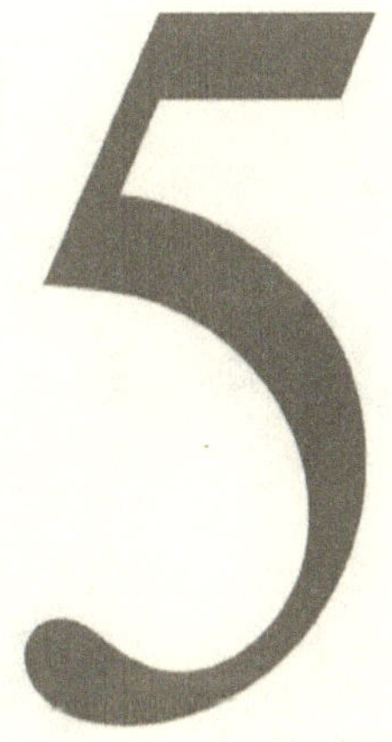



# Tall
# Dance

Jumping Dance

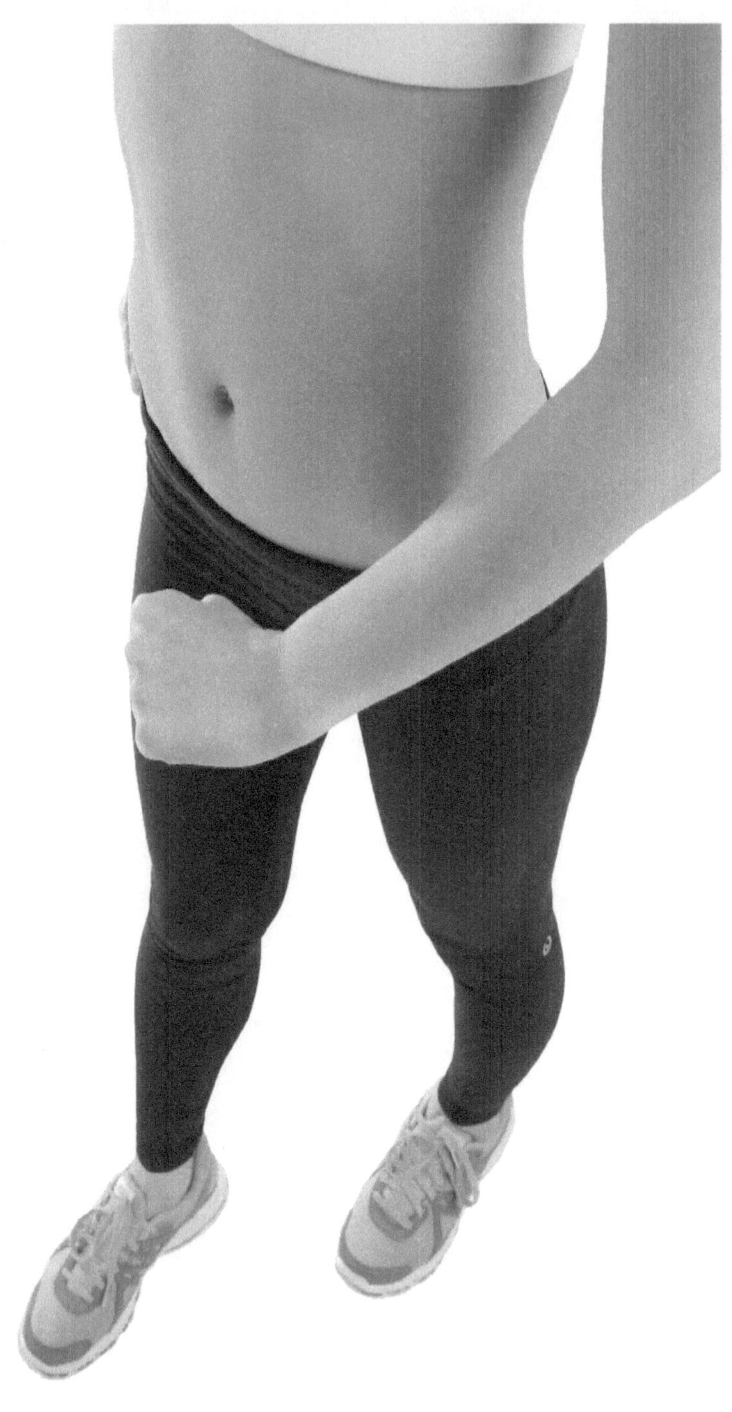

A variety of aerobic exercises help stimulate growth plates, but those are generally boring. I would like to introduce the dance movements that are enjoyable while helpful in getting taller by stimulating growth plates.

# 01

# ROCKCODE
## DANCE

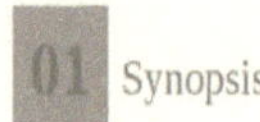 Synopsis

Height could be one of the competitiveness traits in the new generations. Several years ago, there was a great controversy about a woman's inappropriate comment which was 'A short man is like a loser' on the TV program. According to the research 'Height Premium in the Korean Labor Market'(2011) written by Ki Seo Park, an economics professor in Sungshin Women's University and In Jae Lee, an economics professor in Incheon University, 'The wage increases by 1.5% with 1cm increase of height.'

In the cultural atmosphere in Korea, some parents are concerned about their children's height. Height depends on both genetic factors and acquired factors. The genetic factors affect the height 23% and the rest depends on the acquired factors such as living habits - nutrition, exercise, sleep habits -, environmental factors and so on.

The Rockcode Dance is helpful in relieving those concerns from parents because it provides their children with fun and excitement during the exercise that stimulates their growth plates. There is already a great deal of information on exercises related with the stimulation of the growth plates.

The growth plate refers to a part of the arm and leg bones where length growth occurs. Mostly it is located at the edge of the bones and a cartilaginous plate is placed between the bones. From a fetus, the cartilages have turned into bones and the last part of the cartilages becomes the growth plate. All of the growth plates change into bone during puberty. The growth in height of adolescents stops by the end of puberty.

In some parts of the growth plate, cell division occurs lively and in other parts of the growth plate, grown-up cartilage cells are replaced with bone tissues. The main source of the length growth in the arm and leg bones is the active cell division of cartilage cells occurring in the growth plate.

The cell division of cartilage cells is affected not only by genetic factors but also by proper amount of stimulation of the growth plate, mainly nutrients, and hormone balance. Therefore, there are three important points - providing enough nutrients, balanced hormone secretion, and proper exercise in childhood and adolescent period - in order to reach to the highest growth boundary.

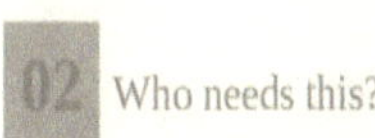

## 02 Who needs this?

The Rockcode Dance is recommended for elementary school students, junior high school students, and high school students who want to grow taller.

## 03 Basic Movement

Place the hands naturally on your sides and jump in place lightly like a bunny. Then stamp the feet lightly as if you are walking. Bend the knees a little bit and jump elastically. Be aware that this movement needs firm contractions of the core muscles because it will help to keep your balance. If children dance can their favorite music, the effect to stimulate their growth plates can be doubled.

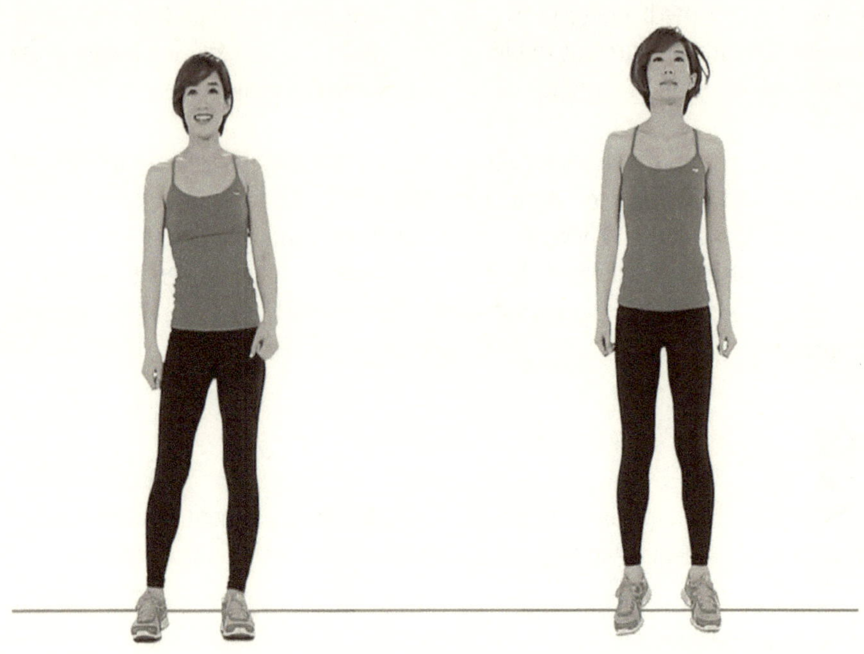

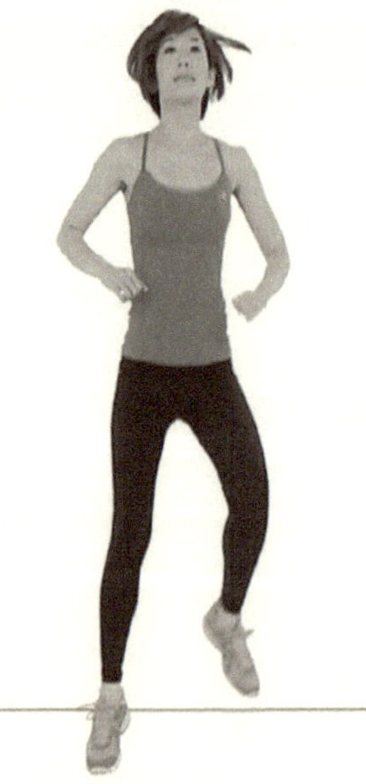

**1** Get into a running pose and jump in place lightly like a bunny.

**2** While naturally getting into the rhythm, gradually start stamping the feet, bouncing up from the floor. Then bending the knees slightly, speed up in jumping. During your workout, it is important to jump elastically as if there are springs underneath your shoes. Be sure to give firm contractions in the core muscles to keep your balance.

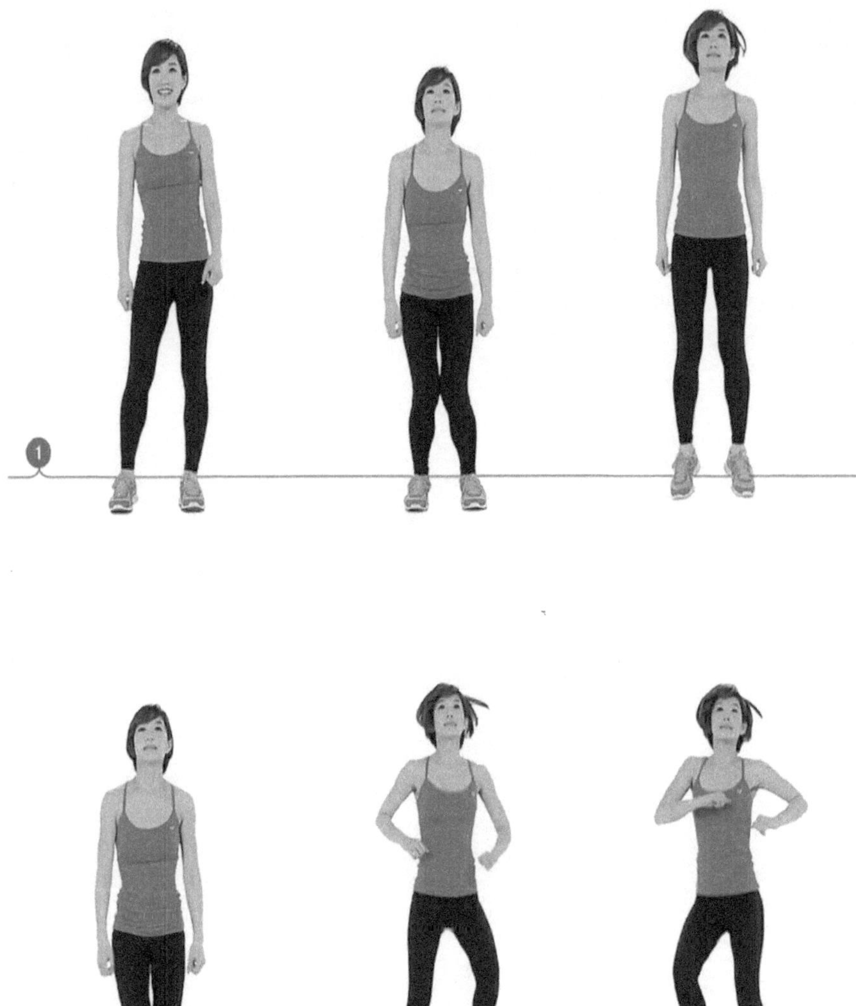

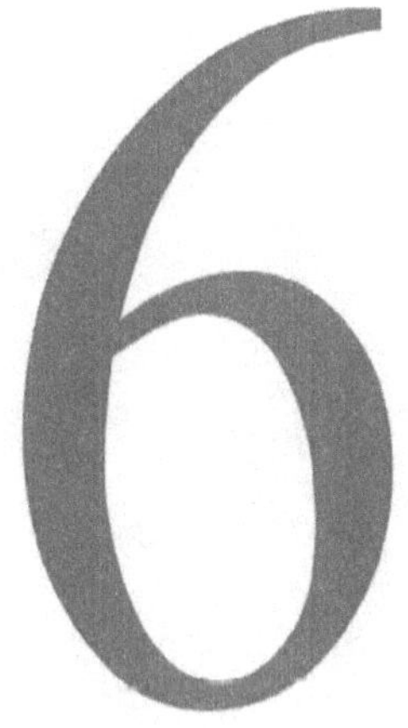



# Dance Therapy
## for
# Menopause

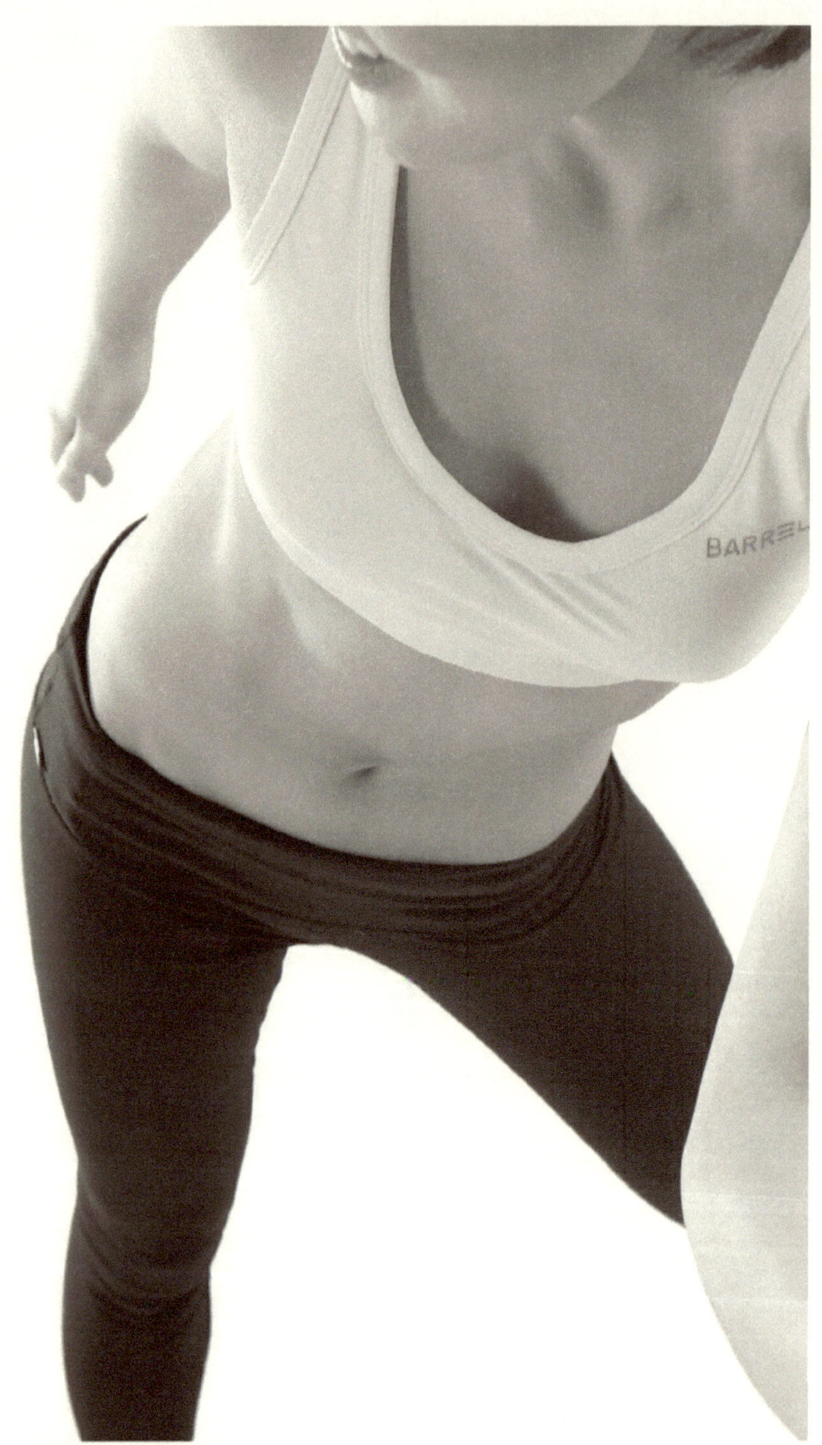

Menopause is an unavoidable consequence of aging, similar to wrinkles on the face. The most important thing for those who have been faced with menopause is exercising. Dancing can be the best exercise to prevent lifestyle diseases and enhance agility, balance etc which tend to deteriorate rapidly during this period.

this dance is an innovative aerobic exercise that does not strain our body, is not limited by place and time, and induces active changes to our body. It can also relieve menopause symptoms like osteoporosis and depression, aligns the spine, and is enjoyable. For these reasons, this dance is the best exercise to overcome menopause.

# 01

# TECHNO

## DANCE

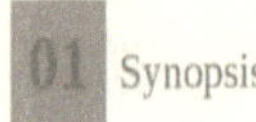 Synopsis

The Techno Dance is very helpful for the spinal joints and it can help align the body. The most important thing in order to overcome menopause symptoms is exercising because it revitalizes the aging body. In this regard, the Techno Dance can be the best exercise for those who have aging symptoms.

**02 Basic Movement**

Push the pelvis forward slightly and without taking it back, push it side to side. Keep the knees straight. While pushing the pelvis, strongly turn the upper body in the direction of the pelvic movement and also turn the neck and eyes to the same direction.

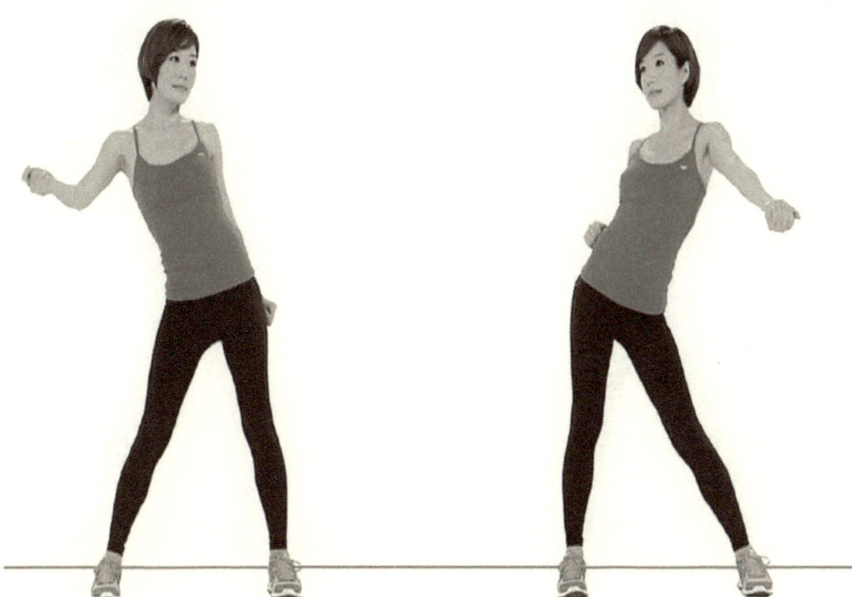



1 Hold the core tight to prevent the buttocks from falling back and place the center of gravity slightly backward. Sway the pelvis to the left while bringing the left arm behind the back and pushing the right arm forward.

2 Sway the pelvis to the right while changing the positions of left and right arm.

3 Strongly turn the upper body and the neck in the direction of the pelvic movement. If you are dizzy, do not turn the neck and keep the eyes looking forward, or move the neck slightly.

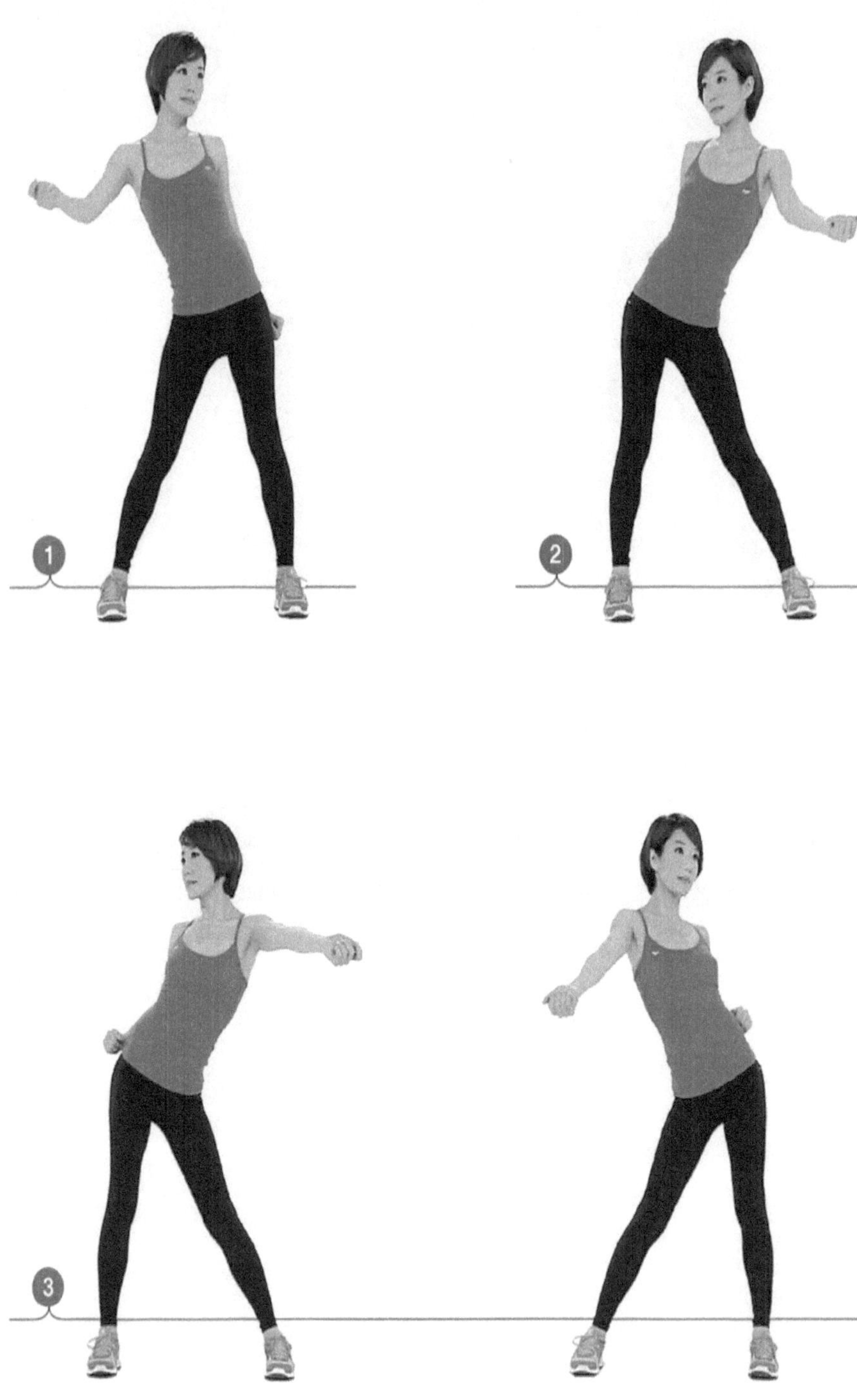

4 When you can dance to the rhythm well, repeat the movement 3 times with your hand on the wall or partner's shoulder.

5 Get into the rhythm and repeat moving the left and right arm alternately up and down.

⚠ Start slowly at first to prevent strains on your body.

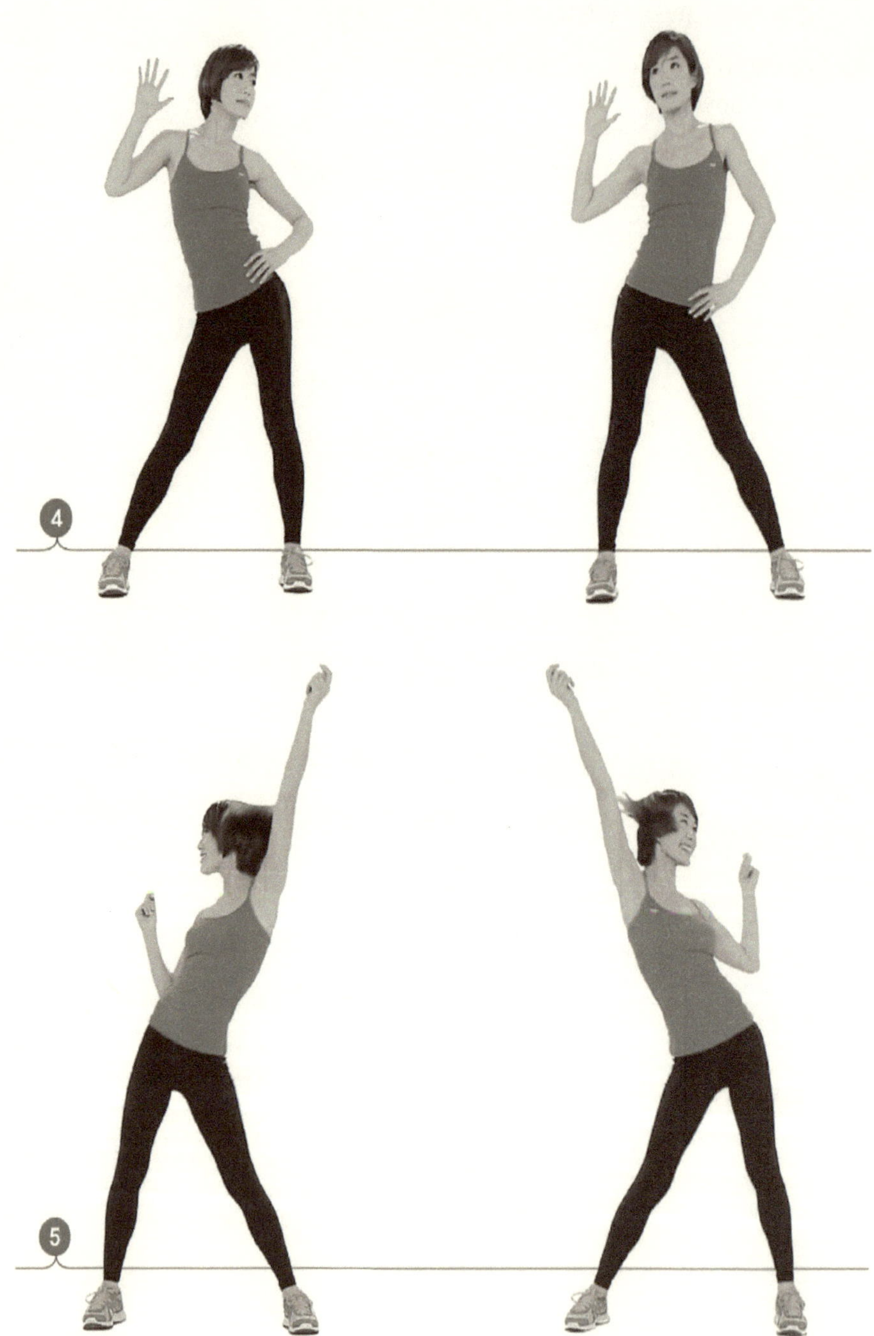
4
5

# 02
# **DOWN**
# DANCE

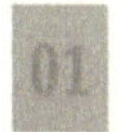 Synopsis

The Down Dance is an easy dance that beginners can follow. It is easy and simple, but very useful for menopause patients who need more energy because this dance is a whole body workout using every muscle.

## 02 Basic Movement

Stand with the back straight and feet shoulder width apart. Then bending the knees and holding the core tight, let the upper body lean back slightly. When straightening the bent knees, raise the upper body. The key is tightening the core in order to keep your balance.

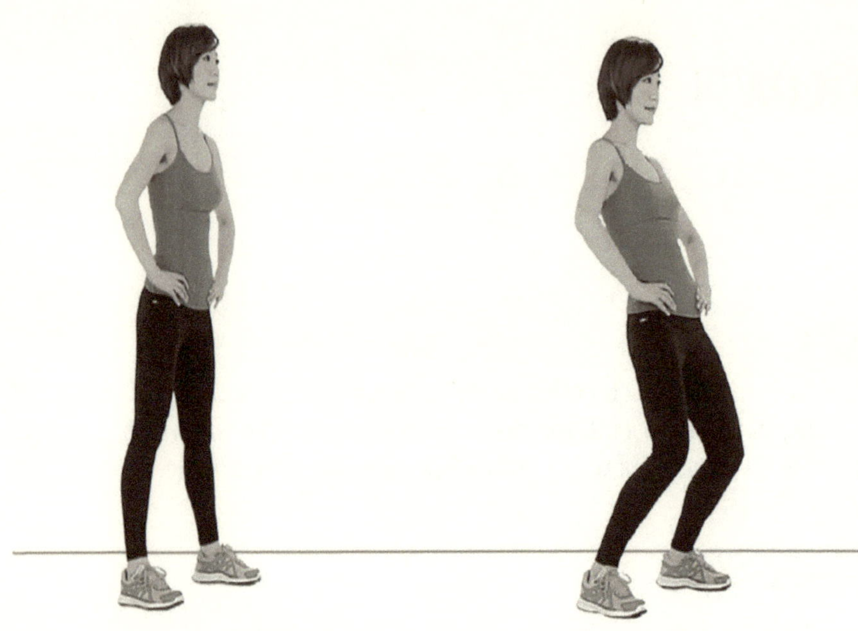

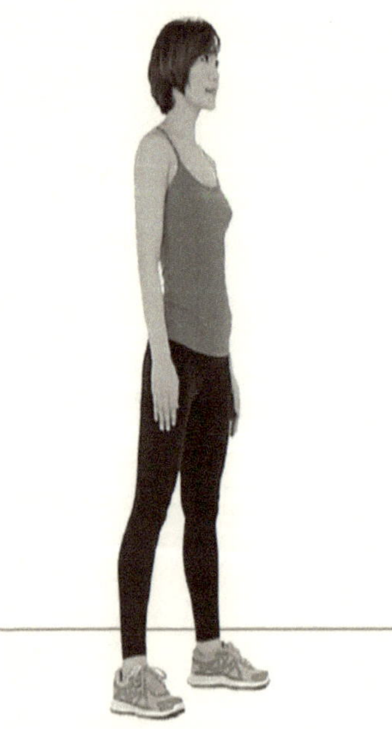

1. Bending the knees slightly, hold the abdominal muscles and the lower body tight to prevent the buttocks from falling back and straighten the upper body.

2. Bending the knees and keeping the core tight, let the upper body lean back slightly.

3. When straightening the bent knees, raise the upper body. Repeat the movement #1~3.

⚠ Start slowly at first to prevent strains on your body.

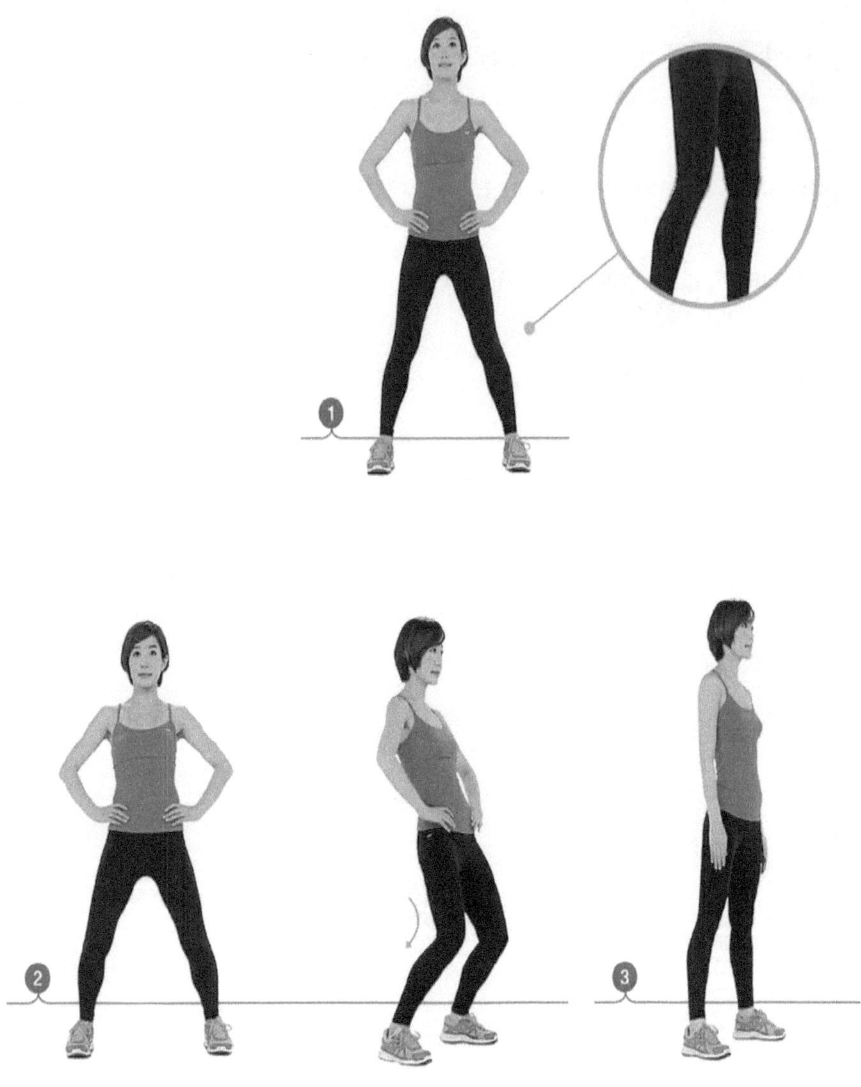

# 7

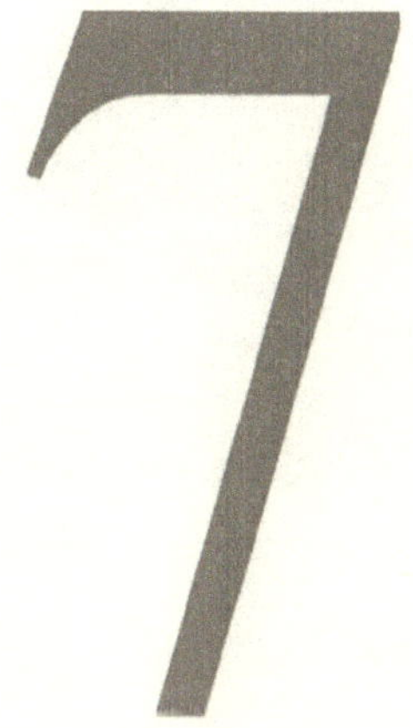



## Shuffle
Dance

Cardiopulmonary Function
Strengthening Dance

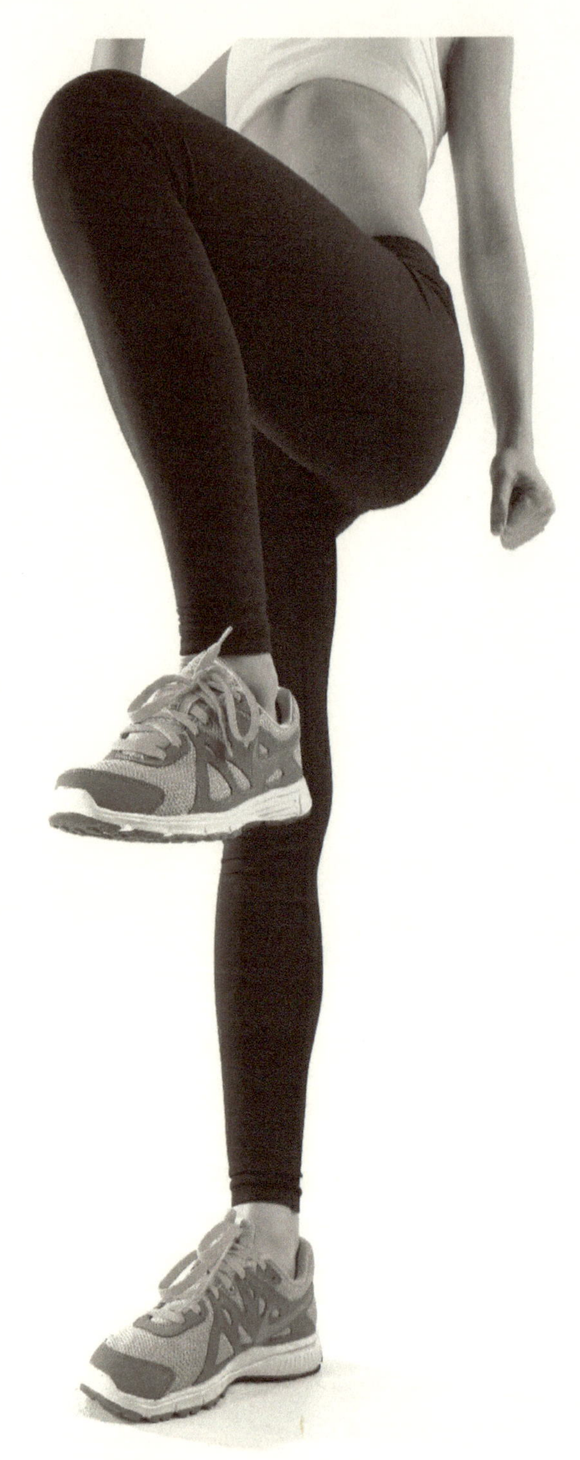

Cardiopulmonary function is the function of breathing and circulating systems that is indispensable for human beings. To maintain life, human beings need energy produced by cells. Our body burns substrate to generate energy and uses oxygen to make combustion. Breathing and circulating systems bring oxygen into the body and supply it to every cell. Accordingly, cardiopulmonary function is important in sustaining our life.

The most effective exercises to strengthen cardiopulmonary function are walking and running. I would like to introduce three shuffle dances that have been made with an emphasis on strenghtening cardiopulmonary function: 'Running Man Dance,' 'Walking Man Dance.' and 'Bunny Dance.'

# 01
# **RUNNING**
# **MAN**
# DANCE



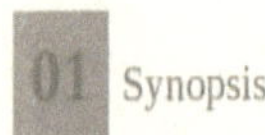 **Synopsis**

Like its name, the Running Man Dance has the same effect of running. However, dancing has an advantage over running in the fact that you don't have to worry about weather or place. Anyone can dance to the music in their home whenever they want to.

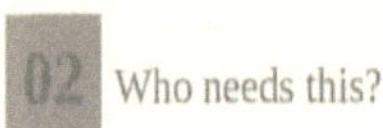 Who needs this?

This dance can be a useful exercise for those who have a weak cardiopulmonary function, who are trying to improve their cardiopulmonary function, or who need to run.

**03 Basic Movement**

When lifting up one knee (right) and straightening the same side leg (right) forward, pull the other leg (left) backward at the same time. After that, pull the other leg (left) forward and lift up the same side knee (left) while you put the front leg (right) back to where it was.

Repeat straightening the lifted leg forward and pull the other leg backward. When you take a step, stretch your chest. Also, as same as walking, pull up your left arm when your right leg goes to the front and pull up your right arm when your left leg goes to the front.

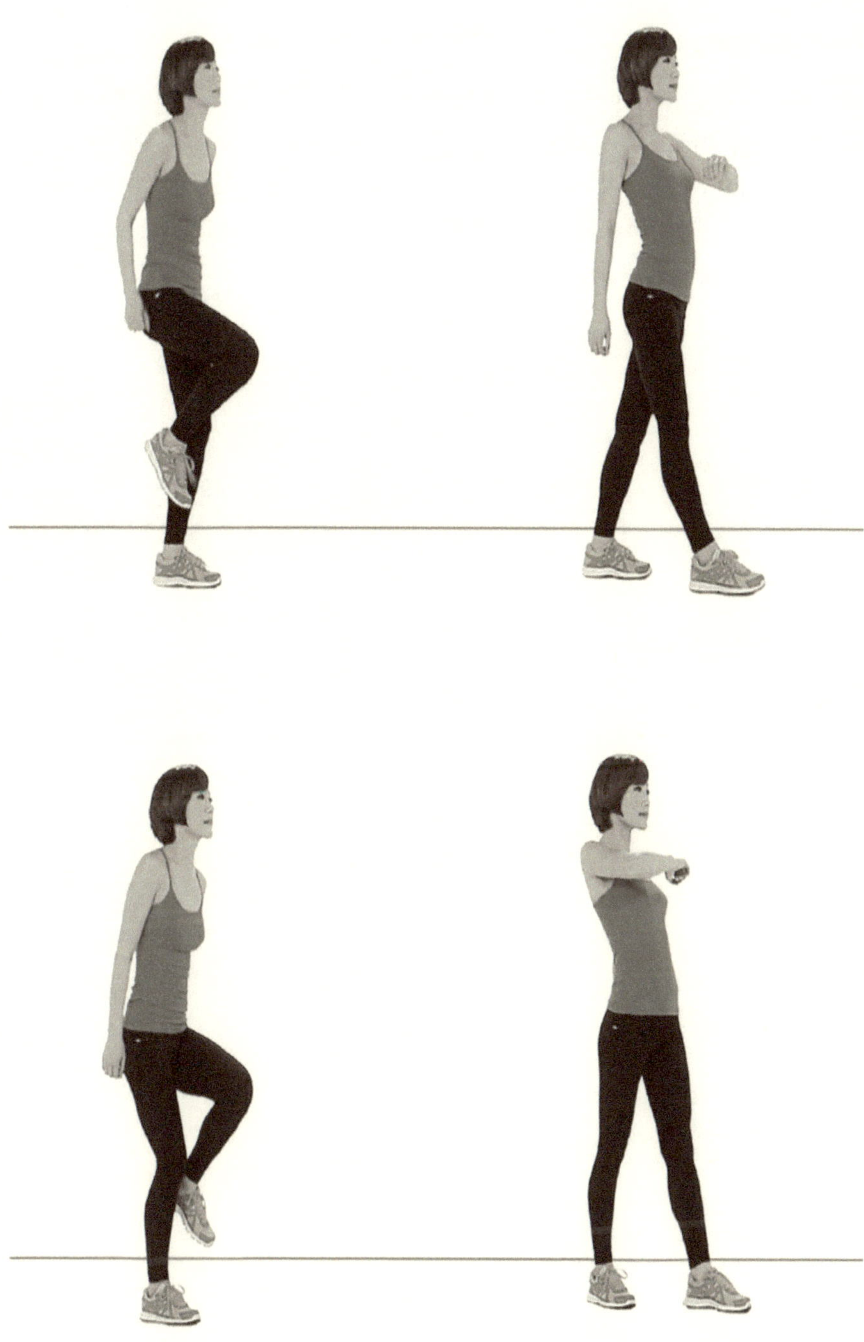

1 Stand with one leg slightly in front of the other.

2 Pull the front leg backward and lift the other leg at the same time.

3 Push the lifted leg forward and move the other leg backward. It seems hard, but you just have to think about 'pushing and pulling' to get you to the rhythm. Repeat the movement #2~3.

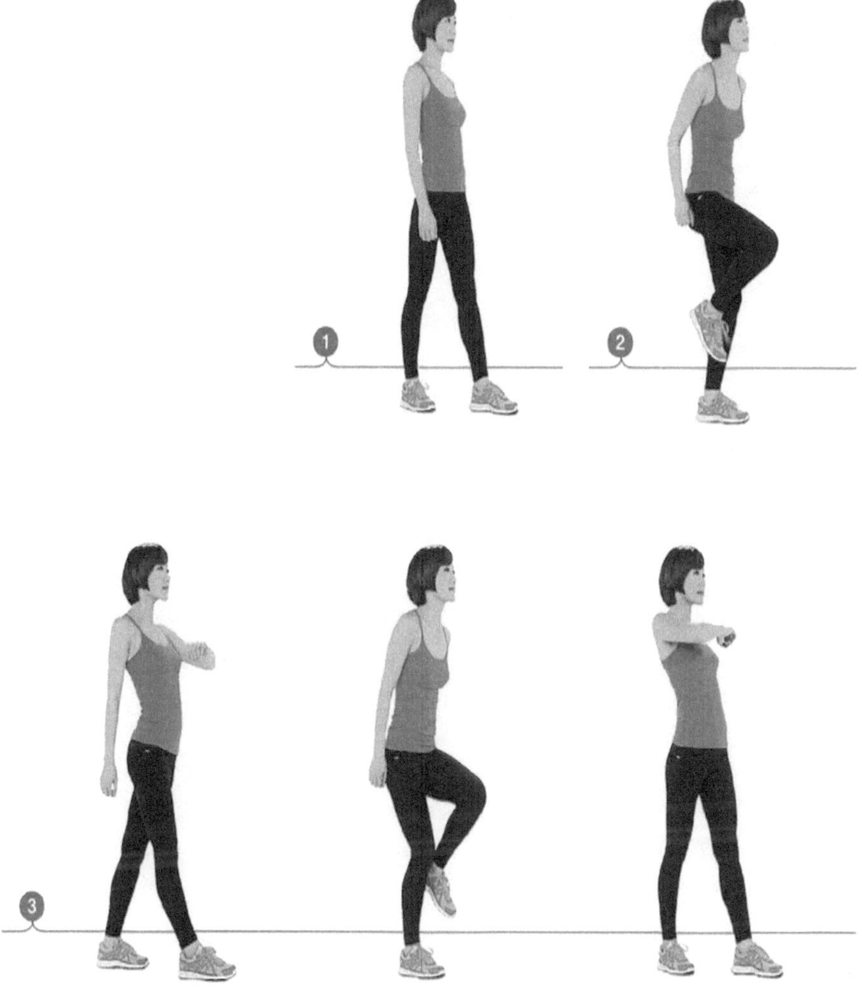
1
2
3

# 02

# WALKING
# MAN
## DANCE

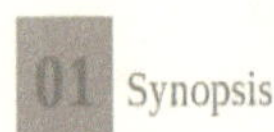 Synopsis

Walking Man Dance, just like its name, is a walking dance. To understand the movements of this dance, think the Running Man Dance with shorter length of strides. If you want to exercise by walking but it is not allowable, then it can be replaced by the Walking Man Dance indoors.

This dance might be thought as less effective than the Running Man Dance, but that is not true. The Running Man Dance can make you short of breath quickly making it difficult to dance for a long time. However, the Walking Man Dance can be continued for a long time with even strides.

If you want to increase the effects of exercise but are physically tired, a minute of the Running Man Dance and another minute of the Walking Man Dance will let you exercise longer and harder and it can increase the overall effectiveness.

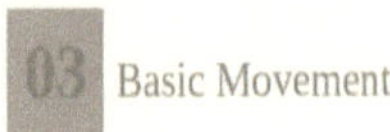 Who needs this?

The dance is for people who want to walk for exercise. Not only people who want to improve their cardiopulmonary function but people who are going on a diet and needs aerobic exercise can use this dance.

03 Basic Movement

March in place as if you are walking on a descending escalator. Walk like you are jogging lightly. Move your arms normally as you are walking.

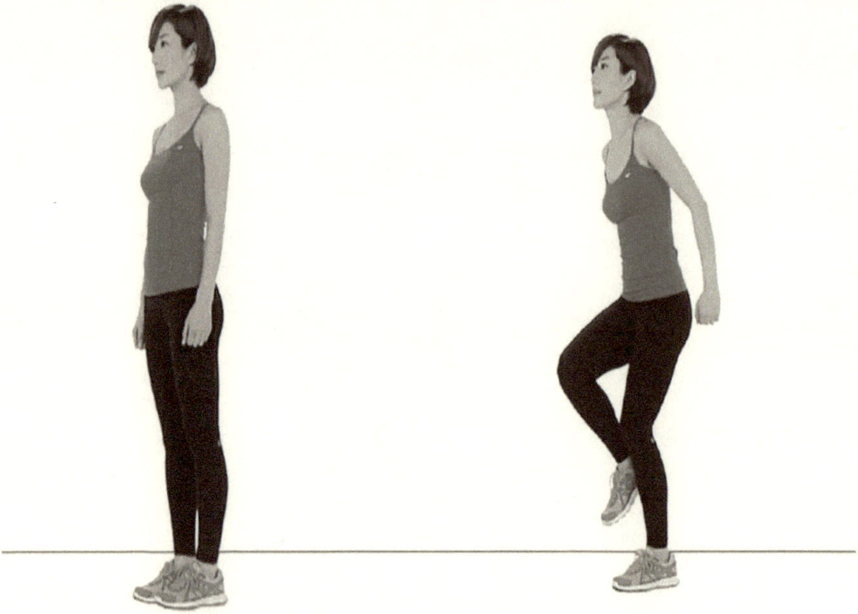

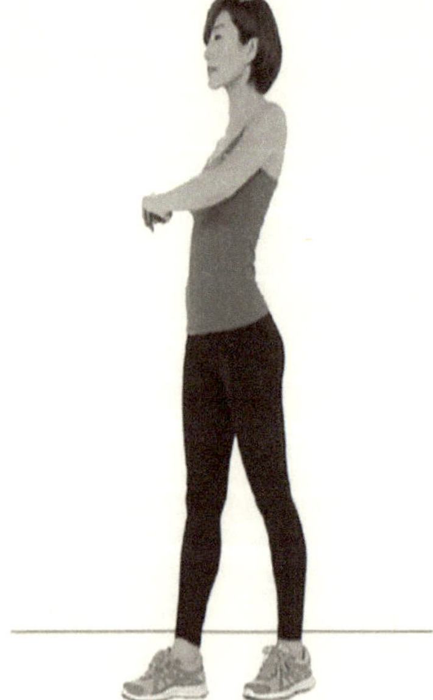

**1** Stand with one leg slightly in front of the other.

**2** Pull the front leg backward and lift the other leg at the same time. The angle of the lifted leg should not be large.

**3** Push the lifted leg forward and move the other leg backward. Repeat walking to the rhythm. This is a smaller version of the Running Man Dance. They have no difference except the Walking Man Dance has shorter length of strides.

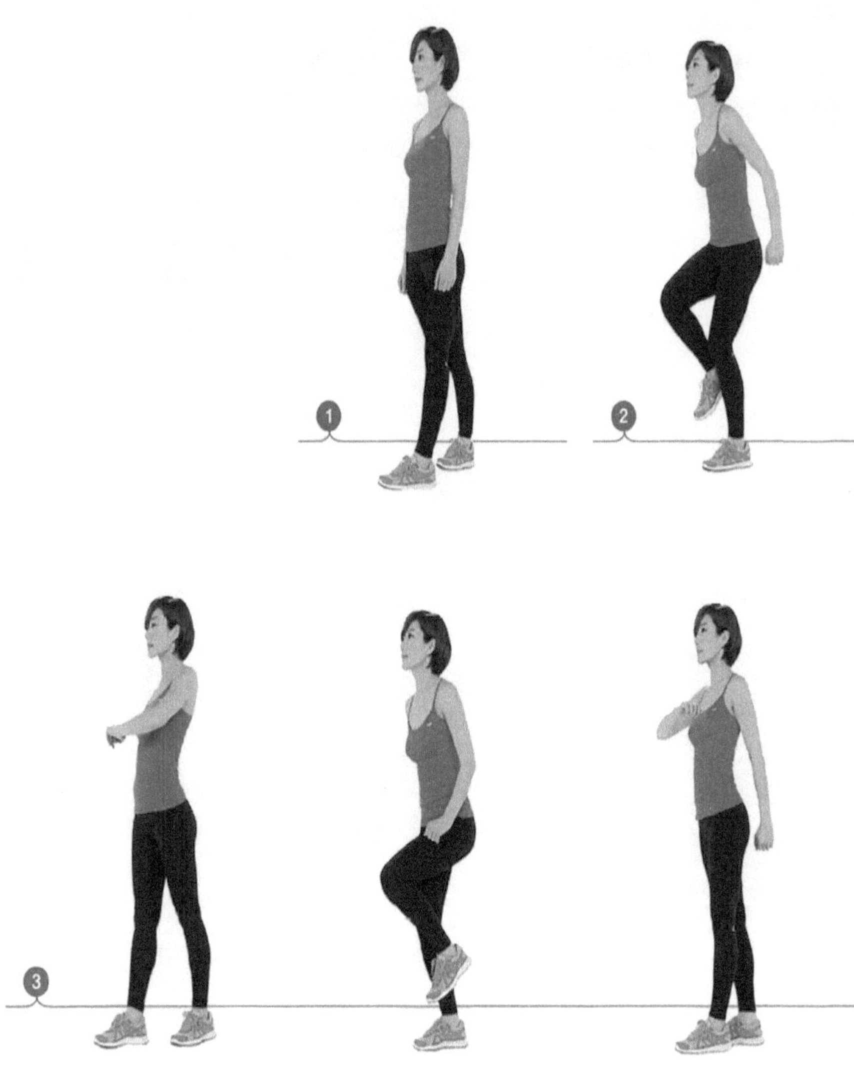

# 03
# **BUNNY**
# DANCE



If the Running Man Dance and the Walking Man Dance are an up rhythm, then the Bunny Dance is a down rhythm. You can understand why it is a down rhythm after you follow the movements. The Bunny Dance is an original version of the Running Man and the Walking Man shuffle dances.

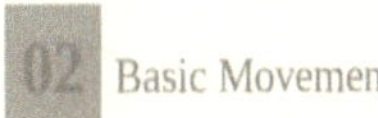

**02** Basic Movement

Lift up one knee and put it down with the knee bent. At the same time, pull the other leg back. After that, pull the back leg forward and lift up the knee while you take a little hop with the opposite leg.
Repeat putting the lifted leg down and pulling the other leg back. Fold the arms to the chest when you lift the knee and put the arms down when you put the leg on the ground. Also, repeat the arm movement.

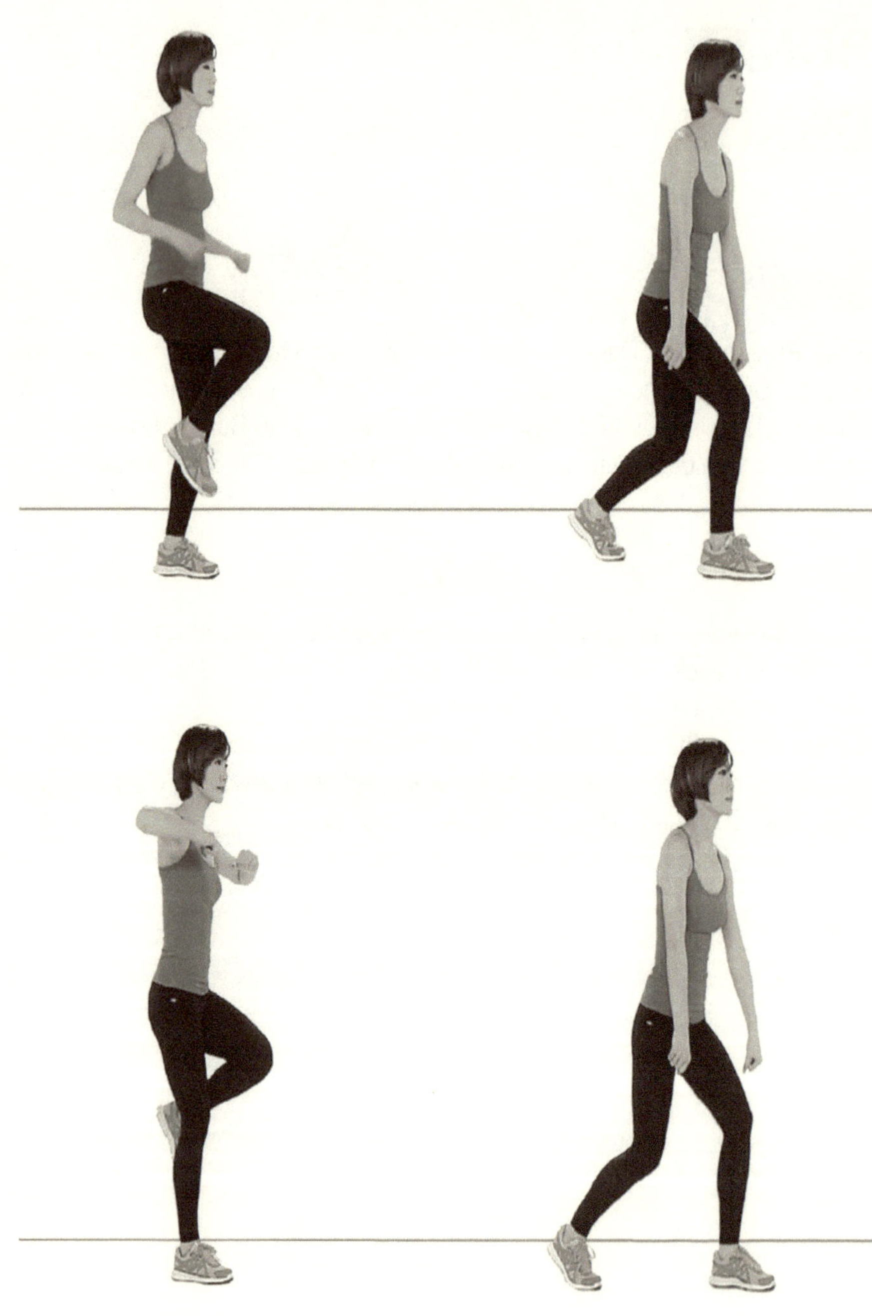

**1** Lift up one knee and raise the arms to the height of about the waist with fists clenched.

**2** Put the lifted leg down and pull the other leg back while pushing down the arms.

**3** Pull the back leg forward and lift up the knee while you take a little hop with the opposite leg and lifting the arms up to the chest.

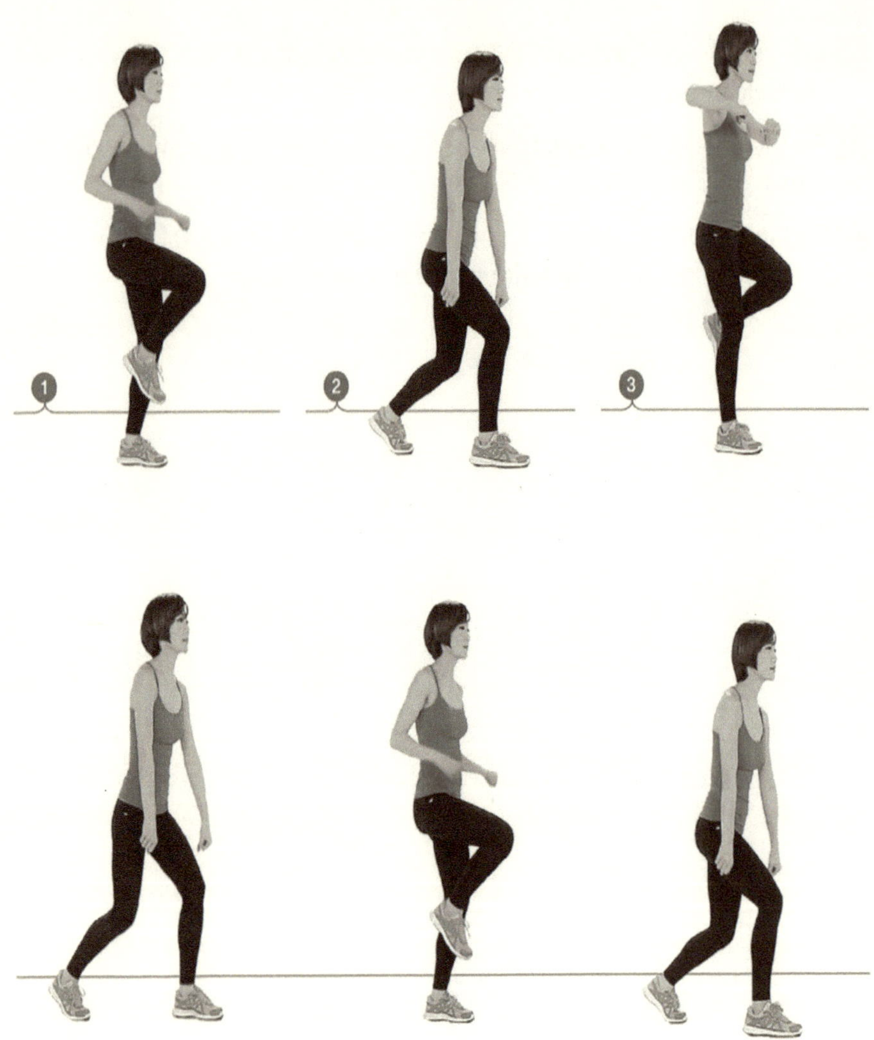

8



# Stretching

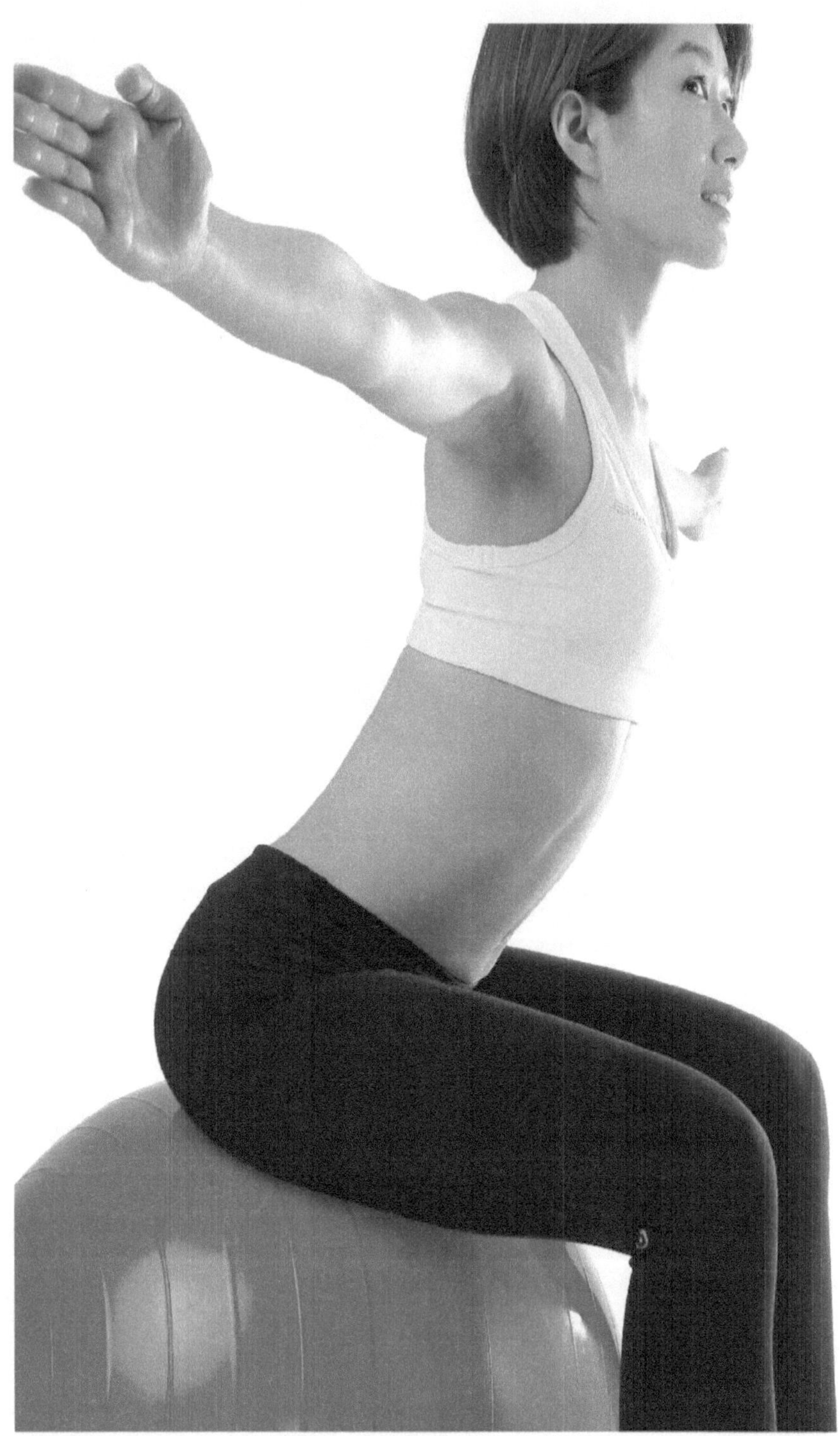

# 01
# WHAT IS STRETCHING?

Stretching is an exercise that stretches the tissues around the joints including the muscles. Generally, stretching is for injury prevention and conditioning for all types of sports through maintaining flexibility and balance of the body, as well as improving the elasticity of muscles and tendons (tissues that connect muscles to bones) and increasing the range of motion of joints.

If you extend the muscles slowly by stretching, the range of motion of joints will be increased due to the flexibility of muscles and tendons. The increased range of motion helps maintain flexibility and balance of the body and it will decrease the shock from external forces and prevent future injury by exercising unused muscles.

In summary, stretching is a very important part of the warm-up and the cool-down in exercises, sports, or dancing because it helps our body to increase flexibility, improve muscular strength, enhance athletic performance, decrease muscle pain, and lessen tension. The most important part in stretching is muscle relaxation, so do not stretch to the point of pain.

There are many different kinds of stretching based on the classification standards. Stretching is mostly categorized by static, ballistic, proprioceptive neuromuscular facilitation (PNF), and dynamic stretch.

Static stretching is the stretching that provides effectiveness through retaining one motion over a period of time. Ballistic stretching is the stretching that uses bouncing movements by elasticity. PNF is the stretching that enhances flexibility of the body by stretching a contracted muscle in the range of motion and it usually requires a partner. Dynamic stretching commonly requires repetitive motions like swing, jumping, and exaggerated movements, but it doesn't use bouncing movements. Moreover, dynamic stretching helps athletes to enhance their performance.

The main purpose of stretching is to recover flexibility by the increased range of motion of joints. Most people who have a sedentary lifestyle usually lack flexibility of the body.

However, it doesn't mean people need to be flexible as much as a rhythmic gymnast or a ballerina. If the body is flexible, exercise performance will be improved and physical demand will decrease. Therefore, it will prevent injuries. For example, this is similar to distinguishing which one is better between two rubber bands of same length and thickness. The rubber band which stretches one more centimeter will produce more force.

Those who have a lot of muscle mass and little flexibility aren't able to produce more power than those who have both flexibility and muscle mass. Flexible people react quickly by a sense of distance and an instantaneous judgment ability in a particular motion such as kicking and throwing ball, so they can double their skills and use them effectively.

stretching is effective to both athletes and ordinary people. If people have great flexibility, it provides general health effects such as increasing the effectiveness of physical activity in daily life, improving body alignment and posture, preventing injuries, reducing muscle pain, preventing low back pain, preventing and relieving muscle spasm, and enhancing the quality of life. Therefore, stretching that increases range of motion and enhances the flexibility is necessary for all activities.

## 02

# STRETCHING
## FOR THE SPINE
## HEALTH DANCE

Unlike other types of exercises, dance can easily cause major and minor injuries because people try to dance in time to fast music but can't control their body properly. I advise you to stretch enough to release neck, shoulders, arms, waist, legs, and ankles before you dance because the exercises require the use of the muscles that you do not use often.

**01** Neck Stretching

**1** Fold the hands together and gently push the chin back with the thumbs.

**2** Put the hands behind the head and slowly flex the head forward.

**3** Using the opposite hand, grasp over the top of the head with fingers resting on the temple and laterally flex the head with a mild force to the side of the raised hand. Repeat on the other side.

**4** Using the opposite hand, grasp over the top of the head with fingers resting on a little behind the temple and flex the head with a mild force toward the diagonal direction. Repeat on the other side.

**5** Rotate the neck slowly in clockwise and counterclockwise directions.

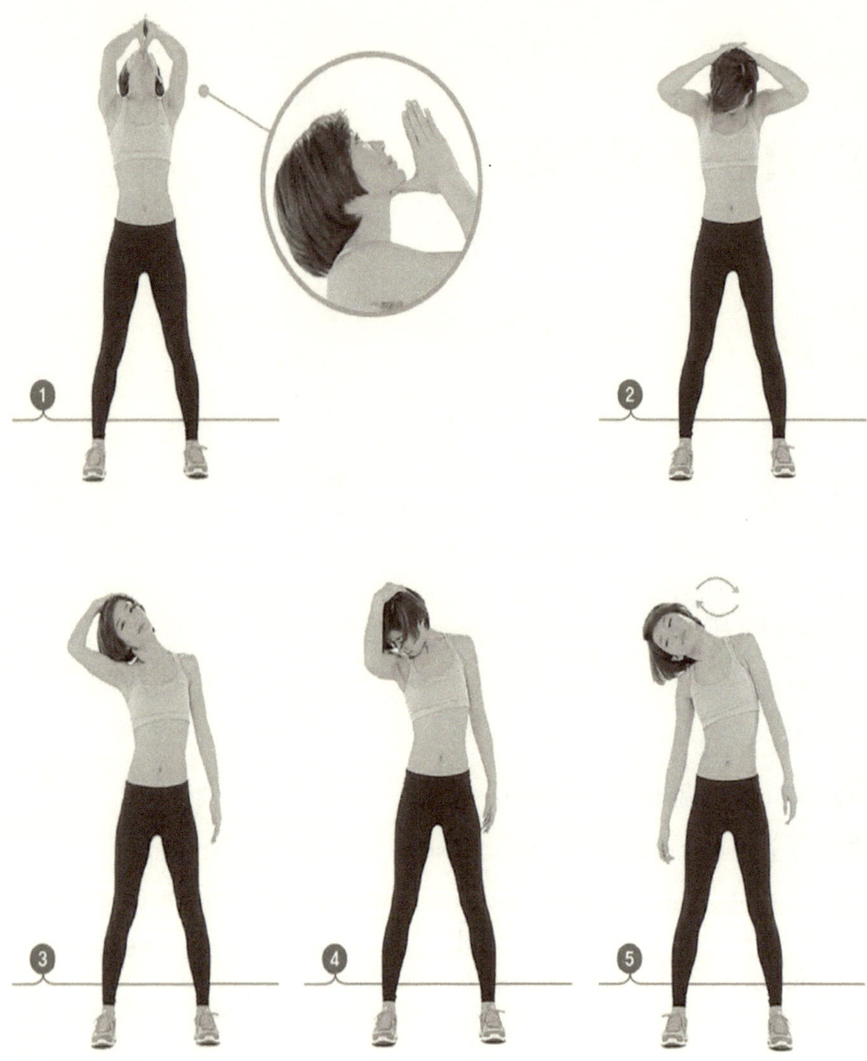



02 Shoulder and Arm Stretching

1 Bring one arm across the body horizontally and hold it with the other arm. Repeat on the other side.

2 Put one arm behind the head and grab the elbow with the other hand. Gently pulling the elbow laterally, lean the upper body to the side. Repeat on the other side.

3 With arms dangling naturally, gently roll the shoulders in a circular motion both in clockwise and counterclockwise directions.

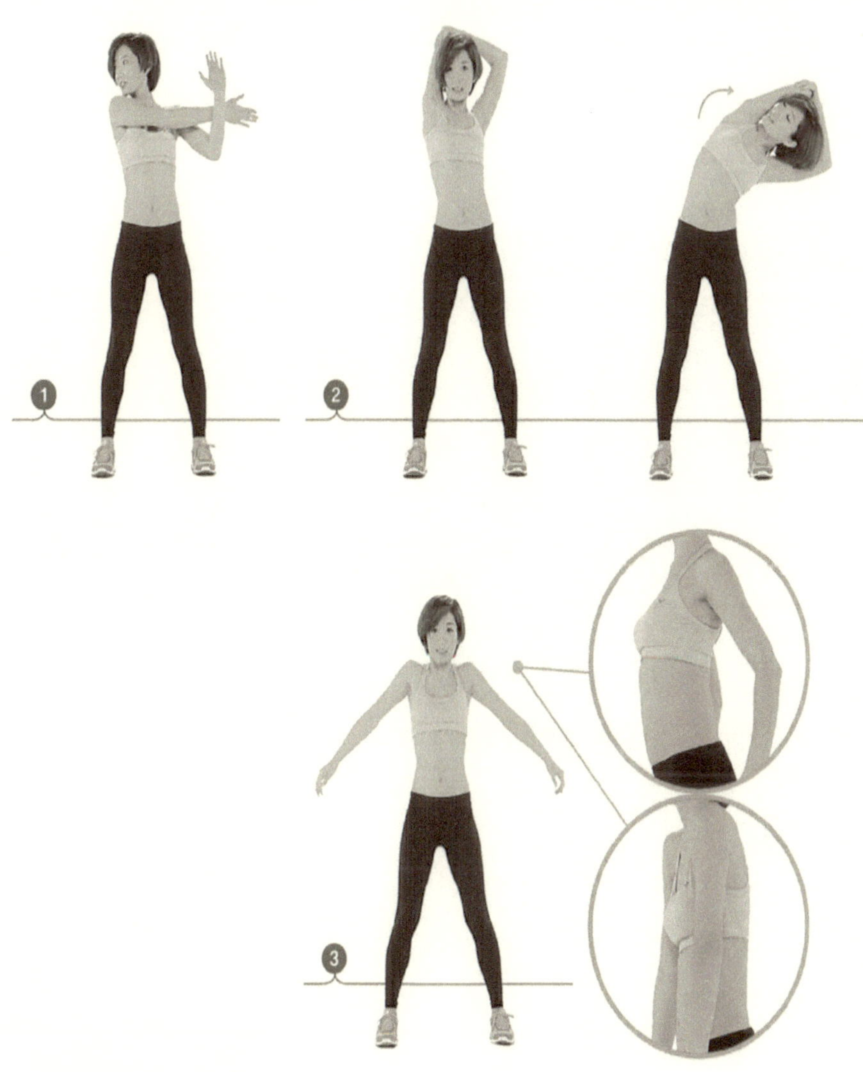





1 Stretch the arms forward and make them round as if you are holding a big ball. While retaining the pose, slowly turn the trunk from left to right and

from right to left. Then move the arms go down and go up slowly. When you move your arms up and down, take your time and do it slowly.

2 Bend the upper body at the waist and make the hands touch the ground. Rebounding lightly will help you touch the ground.

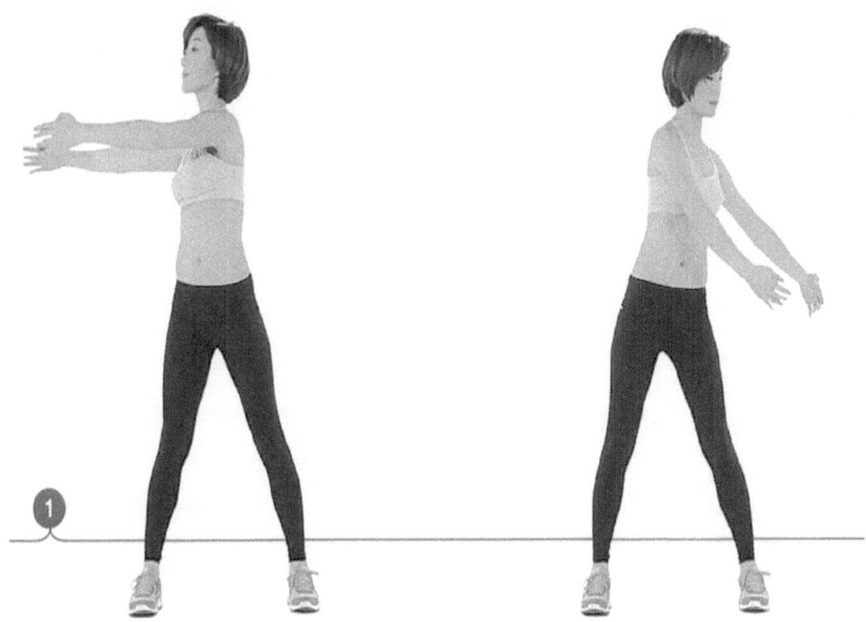

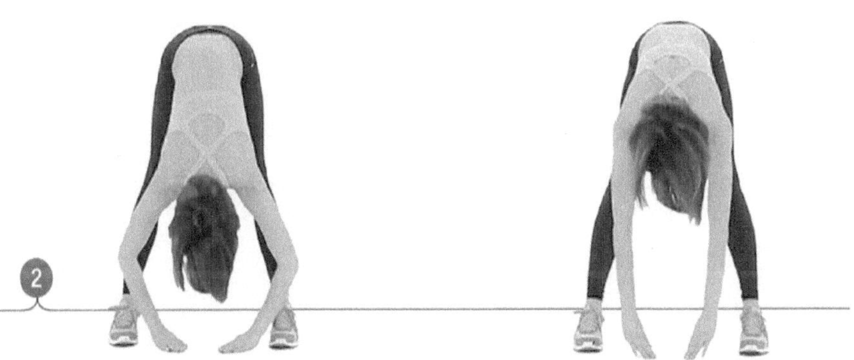

3 Put the hands on the waist and bend the waist backward. Repeat it 1~2 times. (Repeat #2 and #3.)

4 Put the hands on the waist and rotate the trunk in a circle and in both directions.

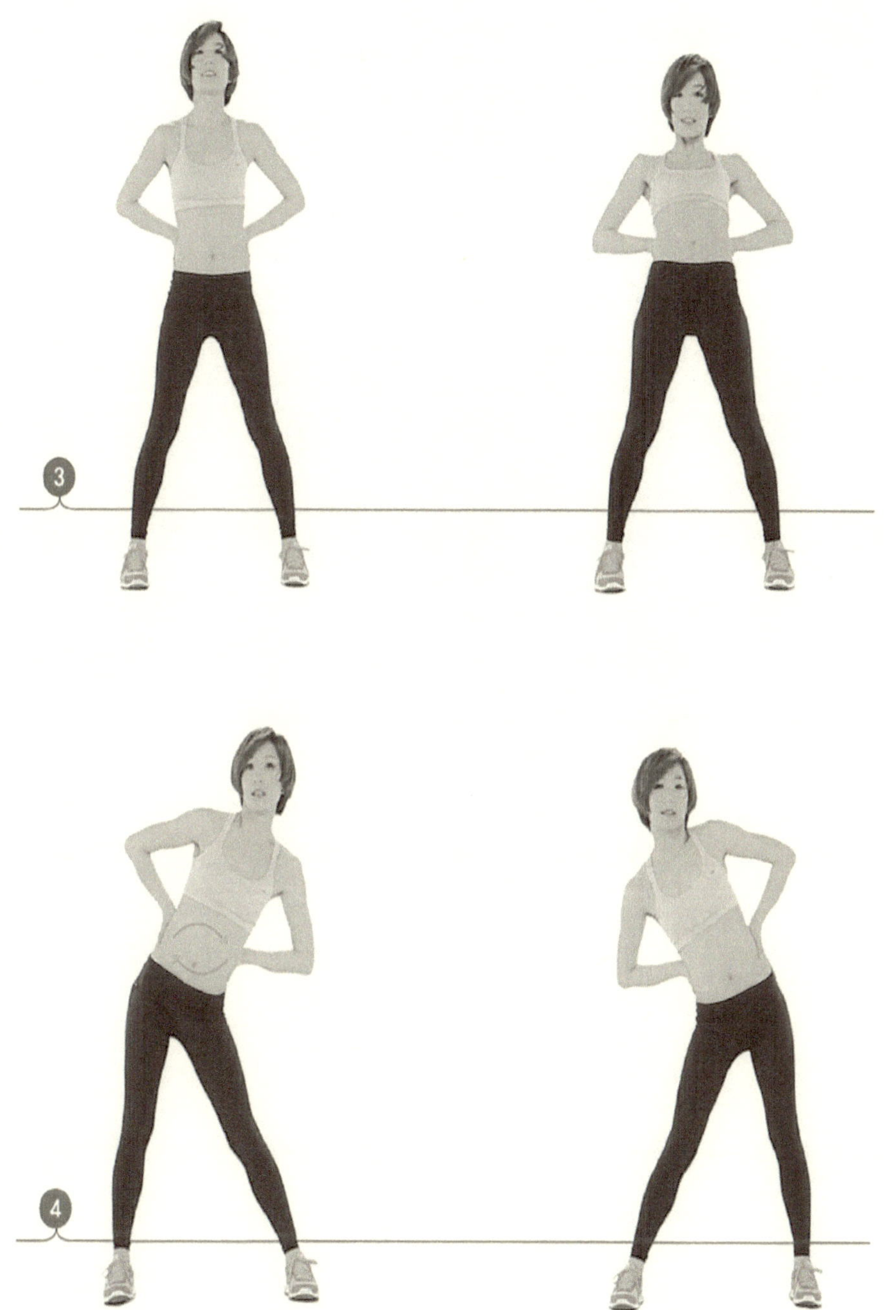
3
4

**1** Put the knees together, place the hands above the knees, and gently rotate the knees in a circle and in both directions.

**2** Stretch out one leg and bend the upper body at the waist. Push down the front leg with the hand. Repeat on other side.

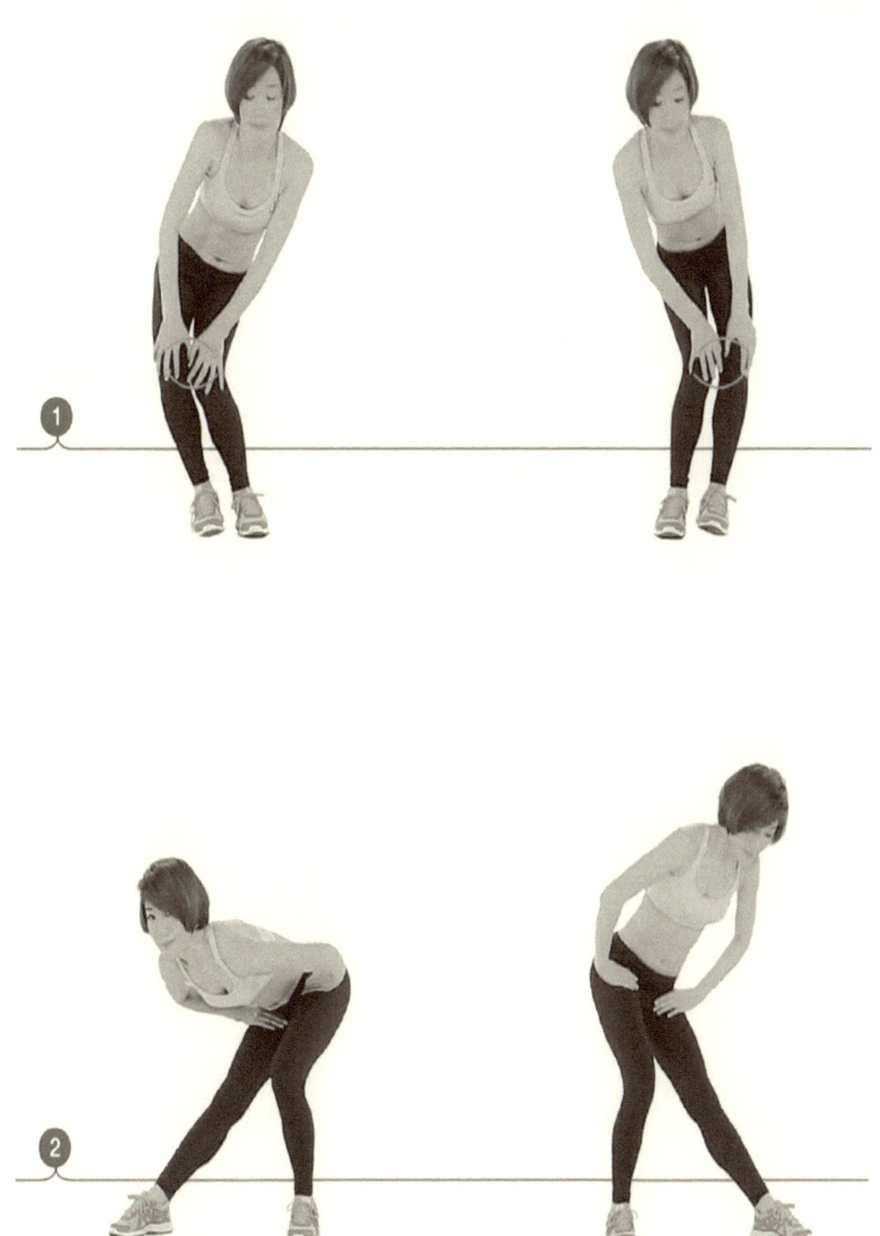

**1 2** Rotate both ankles thoroughly. While rotating the ankles, rotate the wrists together with hands clasped.

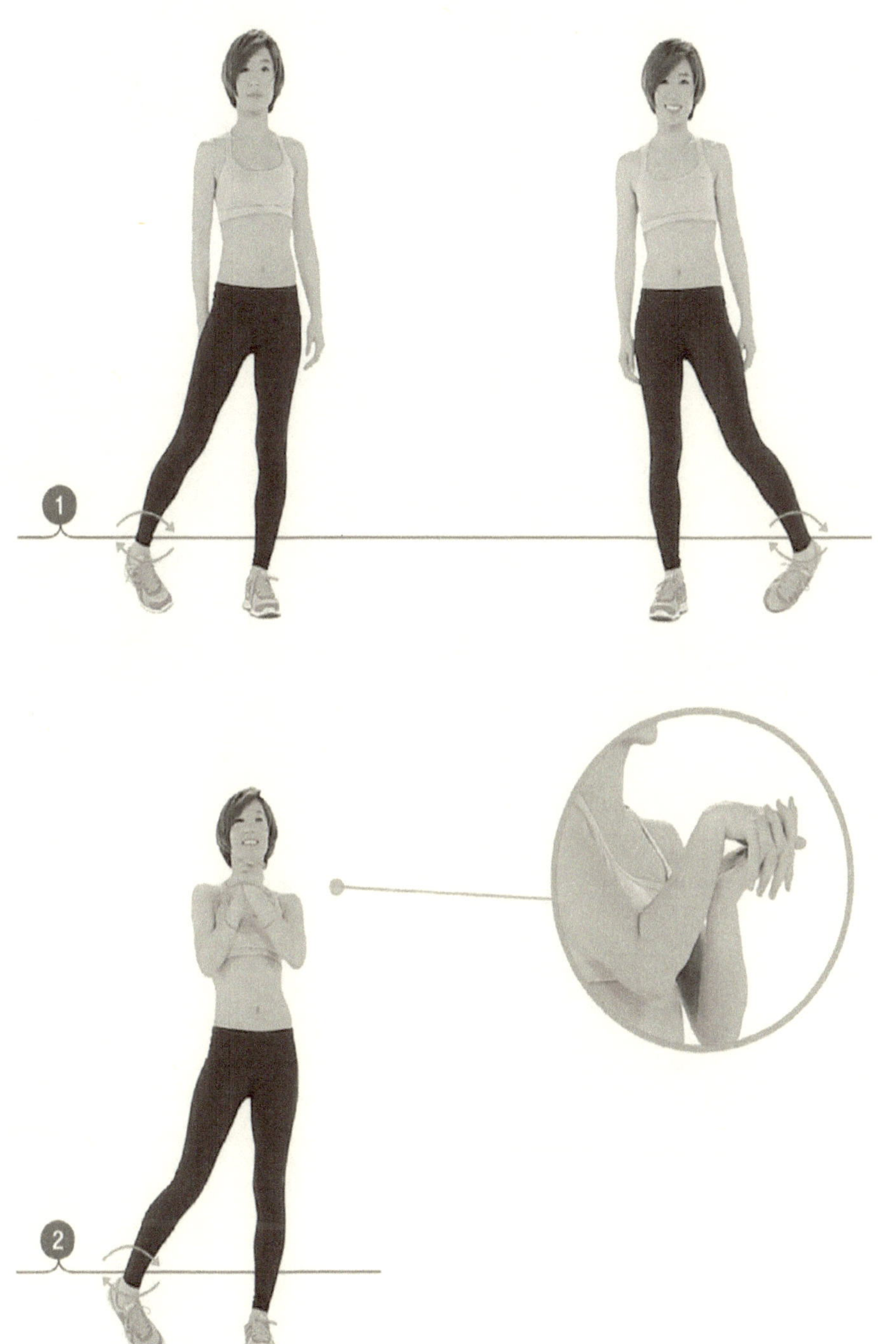
1
2